DEDICATION

To anyone who has ever faced significant challenges or been dealt
seemingly insurmountable odds.

CONTENTS

INTRODUCTION

Some of the names in this story have been changed to protect individual privacy.

I believe personal ownership is the most important skill for any single human being to learn in life. ***I define personal ownership as controlling one's actions, beliefs, and overall direction in life.***

Why is personal ownership the most important skill? I also believe that the greatest temptation in life is to blame something or someone, outside of ourselves, when dealing with a situation that requires us to change ourselves in some way. Blame can also be directed inwardly as we become frustrated with ourselves for the mistakes we make on the road to change. Neither is helpful as neither helps us focus on problem solving. Change of any kind is the hardest thing we do in life as change is often associated with adversity. However, if we are willing to resist the temptation to blame and take ownership by engaging the adversity associated with change, then I think we can experience a greater sense of meaning and personal growth.

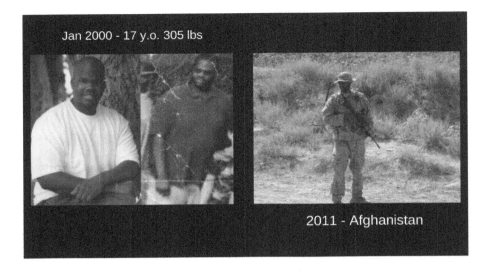

I've navigated some difficult situations in my lifetime: overcoming obesity, getting an engineering degree, getting out of debt, serving in combat etc. I don't claim to be a guru or have all the answers to life's problems but in my experience, the navigation of turbulent situations in order to find peace has always been marked by exercising personal ownership. With personal reflection and time spent trying to convey this idea of personal ownership to others, I've landed on three principles that I believe must be observed in order to practice Personal Ownership:

Action Over Time - *If it's worth having, it's worth fighting for...*

We don't control time. We can't rewind time, fast forward it, pause it, or stop it. However, we can control our focus and how we use our energy relative to time. We can control our actions. Any meaningful goal in life will most likely take a relatively long period of time to accomplish. With significant time comes both adversity and opportunity. The key is to continue to act in the face of adversity so that we are able to reach the opportunity.

Understand Your Story - *Actions are based on beliefs, even when those beliefs are unknown...*

I define the word 'story' as facts weaved together by beliefs/assumptions into a coherent narrative. I believe every human being has unconscious beliefs about how life works. The challenge is learning to recognize when our actions are leading us away from our true desires and doing the work to identify the underlying beliefs/assumptions that led us to taking those actions.

Maintain A Vision - *The process is more important than the products...*

I define a 'vision' as a set of long term goals an individual has for the future. A vision is characterized by being bold, realistic, and holistic. A bold vision forces one to examine themselves regularly. A realistic vision explores the risks associated with pursuing our goals. A holistic vision tries to account for the totality of life. These 3 characteristics produce a process of personal refinement and self-direction that I believe is more important than achieving the goals themselves.

I don't consider these 3 principles nor anything written in this book to be an immutable truth. What I'm presenting is a model that I've found useful for navigating my life and, in particular, challenging parts of life. Maybe you will find some use in this model. I believe that practicing these 3 principles with time can help us find meaning and experience more personal growth even as we face life's most difficult challenges. Life is hard. I hope that these ideas and my story convey to you that we can face any obstacle and know that we have the tools to, Adapt and Overcome.

PART I - TIME

My Mother

I was born in Houston, Texas in the early 80's. My sister was 9 years older than me. My sister's father was a drug dealer and was extremely abusive towards our mother. After being released from federal prison for running drugs across the US-Mexico Border, he lived with my mother and sister for a brief period of time. One night, he narrowly missed hitting my mother in the head with a heavy ash tray that he had hurled across the room in a fit of rage. At that point, my mother was done with him.

My father had been fairly absent from my mother's life. He had been in a committed relationship with my mother and decided to leave her for another woman. Time passed and eventually they hooked up one more time and that's when I was conceived. Obviously, they didn't stay together. Life had been hard on my mother. She grew up with 8 brothers and sisters in a shotgun house in Houston, Texas. Her father (my grandfather) had also been an abusive and harsh man.

When I was born, my mother had become a single mom of two kids whose fathers weren't in the picture. She was strong but when I think about it in hindsight, the loneliness and depression must have been extremely difficult to deal with at times. As a kid, I didn't understand that.

Back then, my mother felt like a dictator. It wasn't uncommon for her to come home from work in the afternoon and begin yelling at my sister and I for the smallest things, like dishes not being done or a toy not being put away. Waiting for her to come home from work always put me on edge as I didn't know what kind of mood she would be in that day.

The weekend was less tense. As Saturday morning gave way to the afternoon, there were many times where my mother would sit by herself in the living room listening to music. She'd be smoking a cigarette and drinking. She would say, "Come here and give me a hug!" I could smell the alcohol on her breath. She loved my sister and I. That was always clear to me. However, even as a 6 year old kid, I could tell she was struggling. Then, I didn't know why she was so angry, or why she was so sad sometimes. I understand now.

I am still not a fan of alcohol. I've always associated it with the lonely image of my mother drinking by herself. I don't want anything to do with the stuff. Besides, I've got my own vices that I'll tell you more about.

As an adult, having had my own share of failures in romance, I can't fully conceptualize how hard it must have been to be the single mother of two kids and neither one of the fathers be present. My mother is my hero. She confronted a difficult situation everyday and she didn't back down. She didn't run. With no fanfare, she worked and she took care of me and my sister. Even more amazing is the fact that she never once uttered a bad word about my father or my sister's father.

Note - To be fair to my father, he has made a huge effort to be in my life since I was a teenager. I haven't done a good job of putting effort into the relationship. I respect my biological father for his persistence and it is on me that we aren't closer.

My Sister

Growing up, my sister was sort of like my idol. I can remember watching her in high school and seeing how little she studied. She still made good grades. She was literally the smartest person that I have ever known. She would draw beautiful free-hand pencil drawings. She spoke fluent Spanish. She scored almost perfect scores on her SAT's and was recruited to go to West Point. Her intellectual capacity was something to behold for sure.

My mom and my sister didn't get along. My sister bore the brunt of my mother's frustrations at home. Sometimes my sister would take her frustrations out on me. She could definitely be a bully at times and sometimes her tone towards me had the same feel as our mother's. When my sister turned 16 years old she left home to live with her boyfriend. It broke my heart.

As frustrating as both my mother and sister were at times, I loved both of them and I knew they loved me. Growing up in the home with both of them often meant navigating the world of two people who were under lots of stress. I was walking on eggshells all the time. I took that timid mentality to school with me everyday.

We're Poor

Like many parents, my mother wanted better for my sister and I. I can only imagine how much pressure she felt. Especially given the pervasive nature of the 'American Dream' that would have been prevalent during her youth and into adulthood. My mom was born in 1950 in Houston, TX. She's a baby boomer. Post Great Depression/WWII era, there was the birth of the American Dream: Home ownership, a car, a good paying job, and the nuclear family. My mom didn't have any of this and I think it weighed on her. The interesting thing to look back on is the fact that I didn't care about any of this. As a kid, I just wanted a safe, calm space to be myself. As simple as that sounds, I think it's hard for most people to find or figure out, whether a child or an adult.

My mom believed that the best way for my sister and I not to have to deal with the challenges that she was experiencing was to work hard in school and get a good education. From as young as I can remember, she drilled into my head that I needed to make good grades and she was very explicit about why, "We're Poor! If you want to go to college, you need to get good grades and earn scholarships because I'm not going to have the money to help you pay for it!"

Her concern above everything seemed to be the quality of life that my sister and I would experience as adults. She seemed determined to give us a fighting chance and the way to do that was giving us the truth of our situation as best she understood it.

'We're Poor! We're Poor! ...'

I heard it a lot. My mom didn't buy us name brand clothing. We didn't go on vacations. We didn't have a house or a car. We didn't do much. We did have love that I could feel. For the yelling, screaming, and bullying that I felt at home sometimes, I knew that my mother and sister loved me. I loved them and *'being poor'* seemed like something that needed to be fixed so I became determined to change that for my family. If college was the way to success, then I was going to apply myself to get there!

I'm not *'Gifted and Talented'*

One of the things that I find ironic about myself is the fact that I did so well academically but I hated school. This is the power of a strong story. It catalyzes you in ways that would otherwise feel impossible. My mother gave me the story that we were poor. I added the idea that it was my job to fix that poverty. And society would add on its ideas about success...

When I entered the first grade I was placed in what was called *'The Gifted and Talented'* Program (GT). It was for the smart kids. Truth be told, I don't remember how I was placed into this group. My mom worked at the school as an administrative assistant and I think she might have pulled some strings to get me in. After all, my sister was a certified genius, so she probably felt I was going to be the same way. Well, I wasn't. But I had been given a title that in my mind reflected a golden ticket to success. *Gifted and Talented* meant that I was smart and I was going to be something. If I lost that title, what would I end up becoming: Broke and Poor? I couldn't have that, so I had to succeed.

The most challenging part of the GT curriculum that I can remember was the reading comprehension aspect. We had to read short stories and then answer questions about the stories. I was a very slow reader growing up and I still am. It became pretty apparent to me early on that I couldn't keep up with the other kids. However, I wanted the label *'Gifted and Talented'*, but more importantly, I wanted what I thought the label meant: guaranteed success, ascendance from what I thought was poverty, and a better life for my family. I interpreted the school as saying, *'If you are a gifted and talented kid, you will have a better life.'* If this wasn't the case, why would there be the label *'Gifted and Talented'*?

The challenge was being able to keep up with the pace of the curriculum given my slow reading ability. At 6 years old, the next step in solving this problem was an easy one: I would copy off of the kid sitting next to me. I would read as far as I could but I would keep close tabs on the kid sitting next to me and answer along with them. I would even make a few of my answers different so as not to seem too obvious. I did this for about a week and then I decided to stop. It just didn't feel right. I also wasn't very good at cheating. I was literally leaning back in my chair and peeking over the kid's shoulder who sat next to me. I remember feeling horrible about it. I don't know how often I had heard the words *'don't cheat'* in school, but I do remember thinking, "If I do well, I want it to be because of my own work, not someone else's. If I get kicked out of the program for being too slow, fine. At least I tried."

I stopped cheating and immediately fell behind. I was removed from the Gifted and Talented Program. It was disappointing. It was my first lesson in failure. I could handle failing as long as I gave it my best effort. However, academically, my future was still on the line. I was going to have to make college happen in another way.

Moving

I began applying myself in school. It was hard. I can remember struggling to make all B's on a report card in the 3rd grade. I was a hard working student. I tried my best to pay attention in class and do all my homework. Sitting and paying attention was actually pretty hard for me. It was a struggle to resist the urge to squirm the whole time. As an adult I still struggle with desk work. Somehow I forced myself to do it as a kid.

Eventually my mother would meet my stepfather. By this time my sister had moved out of our apartment. Her and my mother's relationship was pretty rough from what I could tell and my sister seemed to be struggling, but I couldn't tell what she was struggling with. One time I came home from school to my sister walking around the apartment talking to herself. She didn't make any sense. There was a school project I had built that she had destroyed in her manic state. I ran to a neighbor's apartment and they called 911. My sister had taken a bunch of pills and tried to commit suicide. Later she would be diagnosed with bipolar disorder. My sister's mental health would be a lifelong struggle for her.

In 1992 my mother, myself, and my stepfather would leave Houston and move to my stepfather's hometown of Birmingham, Alabama. I still remember the arguing that started that day in the UHaul. Arguing that didn't stop for 7 years. My mom is the most resilient human being I know, but traumatic experiences with people who are supposed to love you the most, make it hard to recognize when someone is actually treating you well. It was as if my mom knew my stepdad was a good man but her history and emotions wouldn't let her settle into it. Hindsight helps me see the situation with compassion and empathy, but at the time it was shocking to see how angry my mother was. I had never heard my stepfather raise his voice. It was jarring when he did.

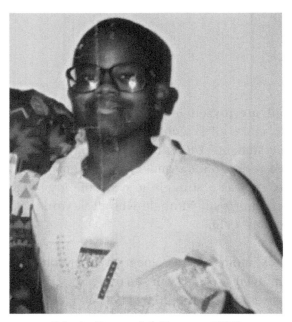

(Me the Day we left Houston 1991)

I can still remember early on in the 10 hour drive, asking my mother if I could get a Yoohoo Chocolate Drink from the cooler. She scolded me for asking. That day, which was already sad in many ways, became a premonition of what was to come during the years I would spend in Birmingham. Constant yelling by my mother. Constant frustration about our situation. Regularly taking her frustrations out on me. My stepfather remained calm most of the time but every now and then he yelled back. Over time, I figured out that he was just defending himself. Either way, it was still going to be walking on eggshells for me.

Once we got to Birmingham and began settling into the new house we were renting, one of the first features I noticed about the city was how many hills it had. Contrast that with a very flat Houston. It was tough just walking up the stairs in front of the house. I was an overweight kid that was taller and much bigger than the kids my age. But, I was timid and very shy. I got teased a lot in school when we were in Houston but our transition to Birmingham was about to take that ridicule to a whole new level, on top of the stress at home.

There was one day in particular that first summer we were in Birmingham before I started the fifth grade. My stepfather was at work and me and my mother were at home alone. There was a convenience store near the house but, in order to reach it, you had to walk through a trail that went through a wooded area and over some railroad tracks. As we were walking through the trees and came into view of the store, there was a group of 5 men standing to the right of us in the clearing. They began cat-calling towards my mother. She just kept walking and told me to do the same. When we got in the store she purchased a few items and she asked the men who were working at the store if they would watch out for us as we walked back through the clearing and into the trees. She also grabbed an old metal pipe to take as protection. As we walked back through, I carried the one bag we had. The men spoke in reference to her body and she threatened them saying that the men in the store were watching and she was prepared to defend herself.

We made it back home. Being 10 years old and never having encountered something like that, I was shaken up. It was scary. In my head I was thinking, "What were these guys thinking of doing to my mother? Would I be able to stop it? Were the men at the store still watching out for us?" When we got back home my mother scolded me. She cussed at me for not saying anything or sticking up for her. She was shaken up and she took it out on me. All I can remember thinking as she was yelling at me was, "I'm so scared! I'm only 10 years old!" Of course, as was usual, I didn't say anything. I just went back to my room when she was done and hung my head in shame. Unfortunately, this was a pattern that my mother would go through. She would be mad at someone or something else and then take it out on me.

As far as school goes, bullying was about to become a bigger challenge than I had ever experienced as I entered the 5th grade. I was accustomed to being teased by other kids when I was in Houston but the intensity increased when we moved to Birmingham. My stepfather actually warned me that it was going to get worse.

He didn't know about how kids had treated me up until that point, but he did know Birmingham and one day he pulled me aside and said, "These kids are different and they may give you some trouble from time to time." I understood what he was saying but, at the same time, I didn't. The reason I bring up the story about the store is because it highlights a pattern that I learned in childhood that I'm still working to unravel as a grown man. When I was a kid, my mom used to tell me to stand up for myself but often she and my sister bullied me at home. I wasn't allowed to talk back in any way and I often found myself as the verbal punching bag for something that I had nothing to do with. So, you can tell me to stand up for myself but when you don't actually allow me to practice that skill I'm going to do what I already know to do. I'm going to be quiet because I was trained to be timid and back down from conflict. As I transitioned into the 5th grade at Carrie A Tuggle Elementary School, I was confronted with that problem head on.

East Thomas

My stepfather recognized I could use some toughness. He knew the kids in my new elementary school were going to be tougher than anything I had dealt with while living with my mother in Houston. I was a big kid and football is a religion in Alabama. He took me to a tryout at a local Pop Warner Football Team. The neighborhood was East Thomas. I still remember the purple and white jersey's. It was still summer time in 1992.

Like I said, I was bigger than the other kids my age. This wasn't uncommon. The age grouping was from 10-12 years old. The maximum body weight for that age category was 140 lbs. I was 10 years old and I weighed 180 lbs. Initially the coaches let me practice with the team as an offensive lineman. I was terrible. The other kids were much stronger and faster than I was. My size only served to slow me down and it made me an easy target for criticism:

'You SORRY!'
'Fatboy, You So Weak, hahaha...'
'You SO Slow!!'
'Damn You Fat and Sorry!'

'You Sorry', was a phrase I heard a lot growing up. It was our version of 'You Suck'.

Practices were rough. I couldn't play in games until I met the weight requirement. Eventually, the coaches decided that instead of practicing with the team, I should run around the field in a trash bag to try to sweat the weight off. This would be my whole practice for about a week. Now I was definitely singled out. It was extremely embarrassing and isolating. I told my stepfather that I didn't want to go anymore.

At that time this experience felt horrible. However, there was one little thing that I held on to from it. One day one of the coaches asked me to get down in a three-point stance and line up against him. This guy was bigger than the other coaches. He looked like he still played football. He hadn't asked anyone else to line up, just me. I was scared but I hit the ground with my three points. He did the same opposite me. His face was serious and I got ready for the snap count to hit. He smiled, stood up, and patted me on the back for not being scared to line up. I was terrified. I had been getting run over by kids smaller than me the whole time. What was this grown man going to do to me? The mental victory was satisfying. I didn't know it at the time but by showing up at the practices everyday, I was developing courage. That's why the coach smiled.

The experience as a whole was humiliating but I never let go of that moment with the coach. Every time I lined up during those practices I got beat. In Houston when I would play sports with other kids I got out-ran, out-played, and was embarrassed, often. I always had to hear about it. I'm naturally competitive, so I hated it. I hated losing. I never trash talked back. Why? They were right. I was slow. I dropped easy catches. Missed easy shots. I struck out, all the time. I was always nervous and scared to mess up because I knew I was going to get jumped on for every little mistake I made. The anxiety played a huge factor in my inability to execute when playing sports. The ridicule and constant threat of embarrassment was a tough road to endure but it made me mentally strong in ways I wouldn't realize until later in life.

That moment lining up against the coach was an extension of what I had learned in the Gifted and Talented Program. Even though it sucks, I can take failure as long as I know I tried my best. It's a profound thing to realize at ten years old. I couldn't have given you words for it back then but I felt it. To do my best, always felt like the right way to do things. I never said anything to my stepfather about the practices themselves. I only mentioned not wanting to go once the coaches had me running around the field everyday in a trash bag. It was too humiliating.

I began to realize how uncomfortable I felt in my own skin and how intimidated I was by my peers. It was a horrible feeling. To live in constant fear of being embarrassed or ridiculed in some way. To walk around on eggshells all the time. I wanted to do something about it but I didn't know what...

2 Promises

That year I started 5th grade at Carrie A. Tuggle Elementary School. Some of the same kids who had been at the East Thomas Football Tryouts were also in my class. Of course, I had to hear about how sorry I was and how I quit.

The teasing and bullying I had experienced in Houston seemed insignificant compared to what I immediately began to experience at school in Birmingham. There wasn't a lot of physical bullying. I suppose that my size was intimidating even next to my timid personality. However, the verbal assault was much more aggressive and persistent. Somebody was always calling me fat or ugly or stupid or threatening to beat me up or throwing balled up sheets of paper at me or messing with my food tray at lunch. I had reasoned long ago that my mother had too much to deal with to worry about me getting picked on at school. I learned to just suck it up and try my best to ignore it when it was happening.

I already didn't like school. I didn't like sitting at a desk all day. It was always hard to concentrate and there weren't any subjects that I found particularly interesting. When you add the constant threat of verbal tirade from the other kids, it made paying attention in class tough. I managed. My grades finally started to hit a stride. I saw more A's on my report card than I ever had. I still believed wholeheartedly that I had to do well in school in order to help create a better life for my family. I was still determined, despite the challenges inherent to my school experience. I promised myself that I would keep working hard and eventually be able to do some good things for my parents.

I ended up making a second promise that first year in Birmingham. Tuggle Elementary had a Boy Scout Troop attached to it. I had always wanted to try outdoor activities so I jumped at the opportunity. As the year began, the Troop Leaders organized a barbeque for all the scouts. My mother dropped me off on a Saturday at about noon at the local park where the gathering took place. As I walked towards my Troop Leader he directed me towards a table where we could make our own hotdogs. As I walked towards the table, a much smaller kid, around 5-6 years old, was walking in the same direction and as we got closer he looked up at me and said, "You don't need any food! You're Fat!" His mother was standing nearby. She came over and grabbed him by the arm. She looked at me and, with a look of embarrassment, gave me an apology.

The rest of the day was a blur. I can remember people talking to me and seeing their mouths move but not hearing what they were saying. I was in my head. Then, I didn't recognize it as pain but I was hurting badly. I was tired of feeling bad about myself. I don't think I knew that there was a different way to feel. I had gotten so accustomed to feeling like garbage. *'Feeling good'* was a foreign experience. My mother probably asked me how the day went and I probably told her that everything was fine. That's what I always did. She seemed so stressed and I didn't want to add to her troubles.

In the days that followed I made another promise to myself. I can literally remember saying these words in my head, "I don't care what I have to do, or how long it takes, but I will lose this weight or die trying!" I was tired. Maybe even more interesting is the realization that the adults in my life couldn't save me from what was happening. It was often by engaging in the activities that adults wanted me to do, that I encountered problems. The football coaches couldn't help me. The teachers at school couldn't help me. The scout troop leaders couldn't help me. My parents couldn't help me. My reasoning was simple: Nobody can watch me around other kids 24 hours a day for 7 days a week. Even if they could, once the words are said, they're said. Nobody can fix the hurt feelings except me. "Ain't nobody coming to save you!" Another phrase that ran through my head.

That Christmas I begged my mom to buy me a cheap weight set from Walmart. I had been a big fan of Arnold Swartzenegger and Sylvester Stalone. They looked like they lifted weights. I watched sports on TV and imagined that one day I could be like those athletes and maybe people would respect me more. Maybe my experience would change. Maybe I would actually feel good about myself for a change... whatever that meant.

That year at Christmas, I got one of those Joe Weider sets with sand-filled plastic weights. I didn't know anything about strength training. It was going to be a trial and error process. I was determined and I had made a promise to myself. Realistically, I didn't see myself losing much weight until I was much older, like in my 30's or 40's. It seemed like such a permanent part of my life. I had no examples of adults in my family who were in good physical shape. Everybody was overweight or heading in that direction. I think this is why I felt it would take so long or potentially not happen at all. I didn't personally know any adult who had managed to stay in good physical shape.

Middle School

It was a rough introduction to Birmingham at Tuggle Elementary but I got through my 5th grade year and I managed to get good grades. When you get good grades in school you get lots of praise. Academics seemed to be the only thing that people celebrated me for and, though I didn't like school, I craved the positive affirmation I was receiving for being a good student. Getting on the honor-roll wasn't an easy process for me. I had to work really hard but the effort I learned to put forth in 5th grade would come in handy in middle school.

William J. Christian Middle School is nestled in a suburb of Birmingham called Roebuck. It was a situation where I had to take a test to get into the school. The middle school I was zoned for would have been a much tougher environment if the introduction I got at the local elementary school was any indicator. Christian Middle was in a more affluent part of town and it was where the *'smart kids'* went... whatever that means. If *'smart'* means learning to stay up all night to finish projects, homework, write papers, and study for tests... then yeah, I was smart. I still didn't qualify to be in class with the gifted and talented kids. Those kids were the smartest of the smart kids.

Life at school was rough at Christian as well. Getting picked on for being ugly and fat while also being bullied into giving my homework to someone else to cheat off of, were common experiences. I don't think it's helpful to go through each thing that happened in this phase of my life. Middle school is challenging for lots of people so I'll give you one example that summarizes the experience:

One day in math class I was minding my own business. The kid that was sitting behind me was a white kid that gave me a lot of grief. He tapped me on the shoulder and asked me to look at a picture he had drawn. It was like a wagon wheel. Similar to this:

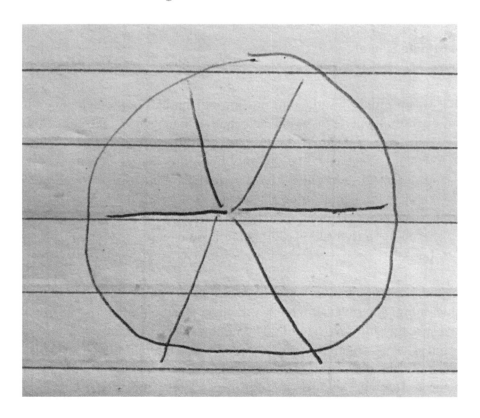

He asked me, "What's this?"
I said, "I don't know."
He replied, "It's what a nigger see's before he dies..."
(The pointed hoods of Ku Klux Klan Members form the center of the wheel)

He laughed and, unfortunately, I tried to laugh with him. That was my defense mechanism. Everything is fine. Everything is okay. What you're saying or doing to me isn't bothering me.

This particular situation was an important one. My dry laugh in response to his joke is an example of all my fears coalescing into one moment:

1. There was the fear of the kid himself and what he represents about Alabama. Based on what I knew of Alabama at the time, when my mother told me that we were moving to Alabama with my stepfather, all I could think about was the movie, Mississippi Burning. It was a movie that was loosely based on the murder of three civil right activists during the Civil Rights Era. The movie had come out in the late 80's and it was my first introduction to racism. I can remember seeing the movie on TV and curling up next to my sister asking her why people would hate us because of our skin color. When my mother told me that we were moving to Birmingham, I immediately thought about the Ku Klux Klan and the imagery of a burning cross in the movie. I thought we were going to be lynched. I was terrified. To have this kid make this joke brought those fears back into the forefront of my mind.

2. Then there was fear of the other black kids. I was one of the biggest kids in the school. Obviously, I am black. The shaming I would have experienced from other black kids if they found out that I let a white kid use the n-word without addressing it directly would have been monumental. I would have been disowned from the race at that moment. The embarrassment would have been off the charts. They would

have called me all kinds of 'punks' and 'bitches'. I had to laugh it off to hide the fact that I was too scared to respond as I was supposed to. I had to keep the situation contained between the two of us.

3. Then there was the fear of what might happen at home if my parents found out. Like I said, my mother always told me to stand up for myself but I had become so easily intimidated by others that it was hard to stand up for any reason.

Easily intimidated. That was me. But on occasion, there would be these moments where something shifted in my mind. They were brief, but they gave me a glimpse of what I could be, if I stopped worrying about what other people thought of me.

38 Points

During PE class we would often play basketball. If I got picked at all to play, it was often last. I was taller and bigger than the other boys in my class, but I could barely get off the ground when I jumped and I didn't seem to have anywhere near the athletic ability that the other boys had. However, one day I was able to do something extraordinary.

I always hustled on the basketball court and I always tried to play the best defense I could. I would work hard to grab rebounds and loose balls. This was my way of trying to be as useful as possible. However, offensively, I wasn't much to look at. I was slow. My dribbling was usually awkward. Shooting was always a struggle and even lay-ups presented a challenge. All this was compounded by the fact that if I made any little mistake, my teammates would jump all over me:

'You Suck!'
'You're Terrible!'

'Damn, you're slow!'

It's one thing to not have a lot of athletic ability to begin with, it's one thing to be a pretty timid kid to begin with, it's one thing to be constantly struggling with awkwardness and anxiety to begin with, but it's compounded when you throw all these things together and people are constantly watching for you to fail so they can pounce on you about it. It's also another thing to be deeply competitive and determined to shut everyone down one day. I was always full of trepidation when I played any sport as a kid but I was always there to win even though my skills hardly ever showed it... my effort and intention were always there.

Then there was this one day in PE class where things clicked...

I was on the court and in the first part of the game another player called a foul on me. This was another kid who I had problems with from time to time. He would call a foul if you touched him a little bit. Meanwhile, I hardly ever called fouls. When I look back, I see how tough I was physically and I was letting people convince me that I wasn't. When that foul was called, I got pissed. In my head I said, "Okay, I'm about to light your team up!"

Up until that day, I had never been seen as a good player. I was someone who evened out the number of people on each team. I was one of those kids who watched a lot from the side lines. But on this day, I was not going to be denied. With all inhibition momentarily being lifted from my mind, I took command. I caught the ball at the 3-point line and drove aggressively to the basket. I shot 3-pointers and made them. Everything was falling for me that day. We generally played 45 minute games that never went beyond 50 points per team. I scored 38 points by myself that day. The final score was 96-94. My team won the game.

No one ever scored as many points as I did that day. I typically didn't have more than 2-4 points in any game that I played in. This was an extreme outlier. The biggest thing that I took away from that day was how for the first time I didn't care what anybody thought about me. I just focused on winning. I didn't care if I made mistakes. I didn't care if people made fun of me. When that kid called that weak foul, all I cared about was winning and that's what I focused on. Everything else disappeared.

Middle school was full of lots of embarrassing moments. Getting punched, slapped, intimidated, belittled, talked about... middle school was also full of lots of studying until late into the night and doing so in a home that was filled with lots of tension and anxiety. But that one day is something that I held on to.

I never saw another performance like that during my time playing sports of any kind in school. However, I always remember that day because it showed me what I could do once I didn't give a damn about people's opinions. The competitive fire I had deep down in me was something that remained a constant theme and driver during the summer when I was trying to lose weight and draw inspiration.

Academics was always the thing that was stressed to me and, because I showed prowess as a student, it was the only thing that was really encouraged. But deep down, I wanted to be an athlete.

Dear Summer

I started working out on Christmas Day of 1992. The Joe Weider weight set I had went up to 100 lbs in total resistance. I can remember putting it together that morning and getting to work right away. It was me against the world. I had something to prove. I had to show my classmates that I was more than the butt of their jokes and the object of their criticisms.

For me the summertime developed a special nostalgia. For many kids the summer represents getting out of school and taking a break: having fun with the other neighborhood kids, seeing your school friends for get-togethers, taking trips or vacations. For me, the summer was a break and a crucible, both at the same time. The end of the school year meant that I could have some time away from the constant anxiety that came from worrying about the torment of the other kids. I often spent summer days at home alone, while my parents worked. No one calling me names. No one embarrassing me. No one pointing out how slow or weak I was. I could think the thoughts I wanted to think. I had the space to dream about being something more and experiencing life in a different way.

Back then there were these fitness shows that aired on the basic cable channels. There were bodybuilders and fitness models that talked you through various routines. I watched them and tried to learn. I also drew inspiration from ESPN Sportscenter. Back then the same episode would play multiple times throughout the day. Watching the athletes and sometimes getting to hear their stories was something that I tried to draw inspiration from.

Looking for the drive to workout was critical because I was thrashing myself. It wasn't uncommon for me to take 3-4 hours to get through the weightlifting routines I made up. I didn't understand physiology or the need to rest and recover. I figured the more I did, the stronger and leaner I would get. At the end of most weightlifting days I would go outside in the heat of the Alabama Summer and run up and down a steep hill we had in the back of the house. To top it off, I would wear a sauna suit the whole time. As I got older, my parents had me start mowing the yard. We had a lot of yard! It would take me 2 days sometimes to get through all of the grass we had. There was our house and we had 2 vacant lots to our left and 1 to our right. Then there was cutting my stepfather's grandmother's yard. All that, and I would still get up early on grass cutting days to get my weightlifting in.

I did this for 7 years. Each year I began the summer with new hope and resolve that this might be the summer that I crack the code. Did I get stronger? Yeah but it was only marginal compared to the physical abilities of the other kids I was in school with. Did I get bigger? Yeah, but I also got fatter as well. Eventually I weighed over 300 lbs in my senior year of high school. If I had to summarize, I would say that the flaws in my approach came down to overtraining, which exacerbated the overeating I was already doing.

From a young age I had learned to deal with the stress of my environment through food. In particular, sugar was my drug of choice. I can clearly remember eating whole packages of Oreos or Chips Ahoy cookies. Devouring package after package of pop tarts. I can remember thinking to myself at times, "I know I need to stop but I can't."

The heavy workouts just made the sugar-carb cravings worse and during that time I really didn't have any guidance on what to do differently. I just figured, if I work as hard as I possibly can and sweat as much as I possibly can, then the weight will eventually come off. It didn't, at least not right away. Getting to the end of each summer and still not seeing any real results was incredibly demoralizing at times, but in no way, shape, or form was I going to stop trying. I couldn't. Just like sugar, working out was a coping mechanism.

It's only with hindsight that I can see this, but working out gave me a place to put the aggression that was building inside me. I think most people you ask who knew me at all during this time, would tell you that I was a pretty nice kid. I definitely had moments where I was being a jerk to another kid but in 12 years of grade school education I was a pretty respectable and compliant kid. With my parents it was the same thing. I didn't cause trouble. I never understood why people gave me such a hard time. I never understood why my mother yelled at me so much. As a grown man with more understanding of my mother's past, I get it. I also now understand that kids are just that, kids. We often don't understand the full ramifications of our words and actions when we're young.

On many days, I can remember just being angry and wanting to hurt someone. Instead, I put that energy into working out, even if it was ineffective. It was a means to exhaust myself and settle myself. It's interesting writing this book after having gone through combat and, now, having fought in an amateur mixed martial arts fight. I've seen so many examples of people who begin engaging in what many would call extreme sports after having endured addiction, abuse, or some other traumatic event. I look back and it makes so much sense why a kid in middle and high school would put forth that kind of effort without much in the way of reward. I was hurting emotionally. Exercising and eating was a way to numb that pain.

New School, Old Problem

In 1996 I started my freshman year at Ramsay High School on the Southside of Birmingham, AL. It was what was known as a magnet school back then. It was a public high school but you had to take a test to get in. I can remember going there in the summer to take the test with other incoming freshmen. There were some recognizable faces from middle school but no one was really a close friend so I felt alone. It wasn't a new feeling but it wasn't pleasant either. I knew things would be more challenging once the upperclassmen were added into the mix.

On the first day of high school I had an encounter that I will never forget. It was lunch time. I was sitting with a group of guys which was a miracle in itself. I had expected to be sitting alone at lunch. It was a good thing that those guys were there because it might have been pretty hard to deal with what happened next, on my own.

Across the lunchroom a girl that I had noticed earlier in the day started walking in my direction. She was pretty and she walked over and sat down next to me. She was also a freshman. She pointed towards another young woman who was sitting at the table she had walked from. This young lady was also very attractive. Immediately I was nervous because I was terrified of girls. I was the fat kid and I had zero confidence when it came to the opposite sex. There are times that I look back on and I can recognize where girls were actually expressing interest in me. However, the story in my mind was that people (girls in particular) found me disgusting. My story of '*Me vs The World*' had skewed reality. What was about to happen next would reinforce that story.

The young lady (let's call her Jasmine) who sat down next to me pointed out the other young woman across the lunchroom (let's call her Tonya). Jasmine told me that Tonya thought I was really cute and wanted me to give her a call after school that day. Jasmine slid me a folded up piece of paper with Tonya's phone number on it. She walked back towards Tonya. I had enough negative interactions with females to know that this was a joke and I had hoped it would end right there. Maybe they would all have a good laugh at the table across the way and be done. Unfortunately, that wasn't the case. Tonya came walking in my direction. She looked upset. As she got close to me she began to loudly cuss me out, drawing the attention of what felt like the entire lunchroom. Tonya told me that I was fat, ugly, and disgusting and I had better not call her or she was going to beat my ass. Of course, I dare not say anything in return. Better to just keep quiet and let the storm pass.

It was surreal like something in a movie. At the same time it made sense to me. This was the type of treatment I had become accustomed to from other kids. In some weird sense it seemed right that the first day of high school, which is such a pivotal point for so many teenagers, would see me have to endure a really humiliating moment. There were other similar moments in that first week of school, not quite as intense. When Tonya walked away I can remember the upperclassmen at the next table looking on and laughing. Thankfully the guys I was sitting with asked me if I was okay. I think they could tell that I was hurt but I did my best to just shrug it off, "I'm good." Later that day after school I can remember looking at myself in the bathroom mirror at home. Would I be ridiculed about that particular incident even more later on? Would those girls taunt me for the rest of my high school career? It didn't matter. I had learned how to look at these things with open arms. While wiping tears from my eyes, I embraced it. I told myself it would make me stronger. To me this was just another thing that I would use to push myself harder and further in life. Why cry, this was a good thing... that perspective kept the hurt and embarrassment from over taking me.

I had become emotionally numb. I was hurting but I never wanted to show it because, In my mind, it meant that they were getting the best of me and I wouldn't allow it. Going to school and carrying on with the mission of getting scholarships to college was too important. I believed from an early age I had to learn how to channel the frustration into useful activities and that is what I did with exercise and academics. The verbal abuse made me mentally tougher with time. I didn't fully realize it then. The frustration and building anger also made me physically tough. At my heaviest point in high school I weighed over 300 pounds. Having limited understanding of exercise back then, I didn't realize the value of stretching. I also didn't understand overtraining and the body's response to continuous stress. I started developing tendonitis in my knees at an early age. Sitting with my knees bent for any length of time was always difficult. Walking up stairs was painful. Long road trips and trips on planes were painful. I got accustomed to pain in its various forms. Toxic stress was a chronic part of life and, unfortunately, school wasn't the only place I experienced it.

The Holidays

The experience I described earlier with my mother and stepfather fighting in the UHaul on the trip from Houston to Birmingham, would be the beginning of a regular pattern of fighting. It had a rhythm that went something like this:

1. My mother is yelling and yelling and eventually crying and yelling
2. Sometimes my Stepfather would have an angry outburst in return but that was rare. For the most part he just took it

3. He might leave the house or stay and inevitably I would be left wondering whether or not it was safe for me to move around the house… life on eggshells

The Christmas season was a rough time in particular. I think my mom had this story in her head of what the ideal life and ideal holidays would look like in Birmingham. As far as I can tell, we never came close to that ideal picture, whatever it was. The yelling that I could make sense of was almost always about money. To be fair to my mother, she had been a single mom to two kids. Food stamps had been a part of our reality in Houston and I suppose she was looking for some sort of mammoth change to occur when she moved us with my stepfather. To be fair to my stepfather, he was grinding. He already had two kids and was helping care for his grandmother. He took me on like I was his own. I have lots of respect for both my mother and stepfather.

There was always this palpable tension in our house and it got really heavy during the holidays. My mother was convinced we were poor. She had gone through hell with my father and worse with my sister's father. I think she just wanted something better but she may have been so focused on her ideal picture of better that she couldn't see the high quality human being that my stepfather was.

I dreaded when Christmas rolled around. My stepfather worked in hotel catering. He was always gone working long hours, especially around the holidays. My mother would be sad when he was gone and when he was home they were arguing. Over the years I began to hate Christmas. I liked the time off from school but the holiday could go to hell as far as I was concerned. With time, I also became cynical about my mother and stepfather's relationship. If they were so unhappy, why didn't they just break up? From the outside looking in, they seemed miserable with each other and it was making me miserable.

Of course, my mother's frustration with my stepfather would often spill out on me. She could be critical for no reason. Unfortunately, my response was to grow the story in my head about life being *me against the world'.* I knew my mother and stepfather loved me but they were under intense stress and I couldn't fully see why. What they didn't know (because I would never say anything) is that I was also under intense stress.

My mother asked me throughout my entire school career, "Are the kids at school picking on you?" My mother knew that I was a relatively timid kid. She often described me to other people as a gentle giant. She knew something was probably happening at school but I would never talk about it. I always felt like my parents were dealing with enough stress and to add my school problems wouldn't be helpful. To add to this, my *'me against the world'* story didn't allow for much help. In some ways this story made me incredibly strong and able to withstand tons of stress. In other ways it made me see people in a light that wasn't true. If it's me against the world, then everyone is my enemy, right?

Coping

Working out gave me a way to feel better about myself and it gave me a place to put some of the aggressive energy that was building inside of me. But it wasn't enough. As a kid I didn't know that much of my behavior were forms of coping mechanisms. As I moved into my early teens, the reality of hormones, sexual urges, and the internet would incentivize a new form of coping...

The first time I saw a hard core porn magazine, I was still in Houston. My sister was 16-17 years old and she had moved out to start living with her boyfriend who was 1-2 years older. Of course, they were teenagers and their apartment was a mess. One day my sister had me over to visit and while she and her boyfriend were in the other room, I was out in the living room by myself and among the clutter I saw a picture of a naked woman. I grabbed the magazine and began thumbing through the pages of what I believe was a Hustler Magazine.

I was maybe 9 or 10 years old. I felt a surge of energy through my body. It was intoxicating. At that point, I was hooked.

In Birmingham, we had cable television. HBO, Cinemax, and Showtime were good for showing softcore porn at night. Back then there was also Pay-Per-View Playboy and other porn networks. Nobody talked about these things. I just got told, "Don't look at that stuff!" Masturbation became a regular practice for me. Maybe before we left Houston, but certainly after we got to Birmingham. Pornography was an escape drug. It made me feel better. Combine that with my teenage hormones and some sense that the images on the screen might be the closest I ever get to a woman, and you can see how it became a habitual practice.

As an adult I have had to reconcile with my use of pornography and I have made continuous effort to remove it from my life. The age of the smartphone has made that difficult but I am determined to change. As I've gotten older, it's also been interesting to realize how connected my consumption of sugar is with the consumption of porn. Stress is usually what leads to either. It's been valuable to see the link between stress and the things I use to cope with stress but when I was young I had no awareness of that connection. I was just fighting to change my body and, ultimately, change my experience of life. I was coping and surviving in the meantime.

I Am an Athlete

I have always had a competitive drive. Whatever I choose to do I want to be the best at it. As a young man, academic prowess was always the thing I was celebrated for, but athletics is what I loved. In the summer of 1996 just before my freshman year of high school, I saw Major League Baseball's Home Run Derby during the All Star Break. I thought to myself, "Hit a ball as hard as you can with a bat? I can do that!" If only it were that easy.

Dealing with the limitations of my body relative to athletics was a persistently humbling process. I was always one of the tallest, if not the tallest kid in my grade. Yet while playing basketball, I was always getting outrebounded or jumped over. I was one of the biggest and strongest kids in my grade, yet in football, I was often getting pummeled by smaller kids. We did physical fitness tests and girls would outperform me on running, sit ups, and even pull ups. In hindsight, there's nothing wrong with this, but you have to understand, this is the south in the 90's in the home of SEC College Football. Girls aren't supposed to beat guys. I couldn't do one pull up for a long time. Baseball seemed like something where I might be able to level the playing field but I had underestimated the difficulty of hitting a well thrown baseball. Nevertheless, I was intrigued by what I saw in the Home Run Derby in 1996 and I went after it.

This was one of the first times that I very consciously and strategically went after the process of solving a problem in a more tactical manner. First off, I had no baseball experience but I did have a TV and we had ESPN. I could watch pro baseball and watch what the pros did and try to mimic it. I saved money that my stepfather gave me from cutting grass and I went to Champ's Sporting Goods. I bought a batting tee, a glove, some batting gloves, 6 baseballs, and a softball bat (I didn't know the difference). I also bought clothing line and duct tape. I knew I didn't have access to anything more than the back porch and driveway, in terms of facilities. I had to be able to practice hitting the ball off of the tee but not have the ball fly into a neighboring yard or window. I wrapped the clothing line around the baseball and tied the line around the bottom of the batting tee. I would hit the ball and the line would stop it mid flight. To learn catching, I just tossed the ball up to myself. I tried to absorb as much as I could from TV.

It was October of my freshman year of high school when tryouts came. From the moment I stepped on the field I knew I was way behind everyone else. I didn't possess a strong throwing arm. I couldn't hit a moving baseball to save my life. I couldn't catch a flyball or field a ground ball properly. At one point, one of the other freshmen who was a much better player than myself asked me, "Travis, if you weren't sure you were going to make the team, why did you buy all that stuff?" It was a legit question. It was easy to see that if anyone was going to be cut from the tryouts, I was probably first on the chopping block.

My classmate's question about buying all the gear gave me some pause in the moment. It was a little perplexing at the time. I guess my thought process was, if I really wanted this opportunity to play baseball, then why not do everything in my power to grab it. Doesn't that make sense? It made sense to me at least.

The tryouts went on for about two weeks. I continued to struggle and I knew that any day I could be dismissed by the coaches. At one point, another one of my freshman classmates, another young woman who was very attractive, said to me in class, "Why are you trying out for the Baseball Team? I heard you're terrible!" It was another one of those moments where I believed I had to hide my true feelings. I knew I wasn't doing well but I didn't realize that I was so bad that other people were talking about it during the school day. In my head I said, "You aren't even there and you know that I'm not going to make it?! Am I that bad?!"

Of course, I did what I always did. I simply flashed an awkward smile and tried my best to make my 6 foot 3, 270 lb plus body, get smaller. I didn't want an onslaught of criticism to come at me from those who were sitting nearby. I didn't say anything in response. I hadn't been cut yet. Nobody had. When they announced the final roster of the varsity and junior varsity I was on the JV list. They didn't cut anyone.

When you are a competitive person and you are interested in sports, it's an interesting thing to frequently step onto the field of play and regularly realize that every other player around you has abilities far superior to your own. At that time, almost anything physical meant that I would be at the bottom of the list. In my sophomore year the school would get a track and field team which it hadn't had. I had always wanted to try the shot put and discus throw. Once again I found myself being regularly outperformed by individuals much smaller and, many times, people who put much less effort into the task. In track meets I would go to warm up and the other throwers were often athletes who also played other sports like football, baseball, and basketball. It was so humbling to look at the way they moved in comparison to myself. In my mind, I still had a chance to get a college scholarship playing sports. That had always been my dream, but every time I entered the competitive arena I saw how far out of reach that dream was. "I could still walk-on though...", I would think to myself.

Persistence. That's what was happening during this time. A sort of idealistic, defiant, quiet, persistence. Give me the criticism, the mocking, the pointing and laughing. Give me more of it. It was good for me. It taught me to emphasize action over words. It taught me to work when no one was looking. It taught me a Do-It-Yourself attitude.

When it came to Baseball, it was watching games and trying to mimic what the players were doing. With throwing the shot put and discus, I bought a couple VHS tapes. With weight training it was reading quick articles in fitness magazines when I went to the store with my mother. Part of my lack of ability versus other kids was the fact that other kids had often been playing sports since they were 4 and 5 years old. They were more comfortable in their bodies. I had to play catch up and in my mind that meant I had to find ways to accelerate my learning curve.

I was starting from a deficit in comparison to others and I was looking for ways to close those gaps. I was overweight. I was very timid and I lacked confidence. I hadn't ever played any organized sports until I was 14 years old. But I sincerely wanted to compete and I wanted to win. My mother has used the phrase 'tunnel vision' over the years to describe what I'm like when I get focused on something. I agree. I didn't care about statistical likelihood or the fact that I wasn't anywhere near the ability level of everyone else. This was a matter of personal satisfaction and principles.

I believe it was during that same summer in 1996 that there was an ESPN commercial that featured a skateboarder doing a trick. This was back when ESPN started the X-Games that featured athletes who were skateboarders, snowboarders, and other fringe sports that weren't yet mainstream. In the commercial, the song *'Do It Til You're Satisfied'* by BT Express was playing. 70's era music. One of the lyrics was:

"Go on and do it, do it, do it 'til ya satisfied…"

As I would watch the skateboarder in the commercial I would think about the fact that they were doing something so difficult, risky, and rare… something that may or may not produce money. Something that might cause serious bodily harm…. Yet they did it anyway. Those thoughts combined with those lyrics spoke to me in a real way at that time. I was always looking for inspiration to keep pushing myself. I would always stop and watch the commercial when it came on. I guess it was the reality that there was no outward sign that I should think I would be successful at any sport or at losing weight. However, win or lose, I wasn't going to stop until I was totally satisfied and at peace with my efforts… just like the song said.

Learning How to Lose

Heartbreak is a part of life. Pain is inherent to living. It would behove us all to get more comfortable with it. Though traumatic in many ways, my childhood also taught me how to face adversity with resolve and a commitment to getting better. I worked hard at everything I did. I pushed myself to get better with the tools at my disposal. I worked diligently with that tee-ball setup.

I can remember one particular at bat in a baseball game during my sophomore year. I had spent the whole summer and much time outside of school working on my swing. In this particular game I went up to the plate and I struck out as if I hadn't been doing anything to improve. I think I swung and missed on three straight pitches. The nerves were always built up inside me because I knew I was going to have to hear about it. I was never relaxed during a game. Never. I was always braced for ridicule for an error I might potentially make. After striking out so badly, I came back to the dugout and I couldn't fight back the tears. It was the only time in my childhood where I cried in front of my peers.

It wasn't just the poor showing in the game. It was knowing how hard I was working on my own to improve myself in the areas that mattered to me most. Yes, I was a good student and I made good grades but I really didn't care about that. Academics was all about avoiding poverty. There was no joy there. Exercise and Athletics was about passion. It was crushing to work so hard and put in so much effort and not lose any weight, not get any better on the baseball field, not get any better at any physical activity. It was so painful. When you add on the ever present criticism, it was soul-crushing at times. These times made all that blood, sweat, and tears feel like it was adding up to absolutely nothing. During my career as a high school athlete, I never came close to achieving anything of real consequence. No awards. No honors. Just lots of losing. Lots of watching from the sideline. Lots of disappointment. Lots of embarrassment. Lots of effort that felt pointless on many days.

One day I was on the track practicing my shot put technique. Just like baseball, I was working on my own with equipment that I bought. There was a coach from a different sport who saw me practicing. He was leading another group of athletes through a workout. He thought it was appropriate to berate me in front of the other students for my lack of ability in throwing the shot put. This coach, who had no involvement with the track team, was watching me practice by myself, on my own time, with a shot put that I bought, with my own money. The irony. I was working to get better and this person looked right past it. Out of all people, you would think a coach would recognize the efforts of a young man trying to better himself. In my mind, I literally remember thinking, "Thank You! I needed that fuel for the fire!" I carried on with my practice.

Did it hurt? Yes. However, starting back as early as I can remember, I had learned to take the ridicule and make it a source of strength and determination. Every baseball game that I rode the bench, every track meet where I placed last in the throwing events, and every summer I spent working my butt off to lose weight only to come back to school heavier than before… It was incredibly demoralizing. I never said a word about it. I never complained. Other than that one day crying in the dugout, I never let anyone see how much it hurt. It's cliche', but I learned to channel the pain into my efforts. I learned to convert pain into perseverance. It seemed like the more disappointment I experienced, the more determined to experience some form of success I became. I thought that success was a sports scholarship or being able to walk on to a college sports team of some kind. Success, at that time, actually ended up being something much more simple and personal. Also, much more profound.

The Right Conditions

Senior year in high school was definitely an odd year of school for me. As studious and responsible as I had always been, I really began to run low on academic motivation. Throughout all of middle school and high school I was fully convinced that my only path to a better life was through academic performance and getting to college. At this point I had spent countless nights, up all night studying. I had spent countless hours practicing both baseball and throwing the shot put and discus on my own. I had spent countless hours cutting grass and doing chores. And of course, I had spent countless hours working out on my own to try to lose weight.

The focus on academics was paying off. My GPA was high. I had extracurricular activities to put on my college application, to include participation in JROTC. My JROTC instructor even strongly recommended that I apply to West Point. He felt that I had the sort of self discipline that a person needed to thrive in that environment. I was firmly against it. I had put up with crap from other people for so long. I wasn't about to voluntarily sign up to deal with more yelling and screaming and stress. I was done with other people's garbage treatment: peers, parents, teachers, everybody.

As people were scrambling to apply to this school or that school, I made up my mind that I was only going to apply to one school, The University of Houston. My parents always talked about Houston with great reverence. They felt that there was more opportunity there and that the city was more progressive in terms of race. I saw Houston as a return to something that had been better in my own experience. Remember, the teasing and bullying I experienced seemed to grow to a much greater intensity when we moved from Houston to Birmingham. For me, Birmingham represented a place of intense suffering and frustration. I wanted to leave behind all memories of my time growing up there. I didn't have any strong friendships. In terms of my peer group, I felt like I had no connections worth fighting for in Birmingham. I wanted to start clean in Houston.

Another reason that I only filled out one application was the fact that I was burned out. I was sick of school and sick of people. Every adult is all up in your face about college applications and every senior is freaking out about the application process. I had worked too hard and endured too much crap to spend my senior year freaking out about college. If I got in, fine. If I didn't, fine, whatever. There's a point where you work so hard that the process almost loses meaning and that's where I was with school. I certainly didn't recognize it as burnout and none of the adults in my life would've known because I never talked with anyone about how I was actually feeling. I was always soldiering on. Maybe that's why my JROTC instructor felt I was good West Point material.

Fortunately, UH accepted me and granted me some partial academic scholarships to go along with the deal. If I recall correctly, I had completed all of my application material at the beginning of the second semester of my senior year. Things were generally good. I was ahead on my credit requirements for graduation, so I only had to be at school for half the normal school day. I was working part time, so I had some of my own money and my parents had given me a car the year before.

I had decided to drop baseball my final year and focus on throwing for the track team. I figured if I had any chance to be an athlete in college, it was going to happen as a thrower.

During the first semester I had shown some prowess throwing the discus but I ran into a back injury early on that slowed me down. I was warming up one day and suddenly my back seized up. This injury would come back to visit me later in life and much later I would learn that sometimes people who have experienced lots of trauma carry the memories in their bodies. I didn't have any knowledge of this at the time. As always, I put forth intense effort but I didn't do much with the track team that year. But something else happened... something better.

Being a senior, being at school for half days only, and having my own money and transportation, set the conditions for a shift. The track and field coach had all his athletes get physicals at the beginning of the outdoor season in January of 2000. This, again, was my final semester in school. I got on the scale at the clinic and it read 305 pounds. Despite so much effort over the years I just couldn't seem to get the weight off. I originally thought the back injury was related to my weight. After all, I had chronic tendonitis in my knees. I was always in pain. The track coach also had all of his athletes run a mile or two as a part of our daily warm ups. A week after hitting the scale I decided to weigh myself again. I worked at a Sears Department Store in the local Century Plaza Mall (This Mall Closed Years Ago). On the other end of the mall there was a GNC Store (General Nutrition Centers) that I visited sometimes for protein supplements to aid my workout recovery. They had a scale in front of the store. Out of curiosity, a week after the physical I wanted to get on the scale and see what I weighed. The scale printed out a little piece of paper: 298 pounds.

"Hummm... I lost 7 lbs in a week, huh?"

In reality, I was using a different scale at a different time of the week. However, in my head I didn't register any of that. Whether I actually lost weight or not, in my mind the scale had moved and this was just the little bit of daylight I needed to get on a new path. The conditions were right. Being a senior and having a shorter school day meant that I didn't have to deal with the stress from my classmates the way I did in times past. Less stress meant less stress eating. Having my own transportation and money meant that I could control more of what I bought to eat. Initially, I associated the weight loss with running everyday for warm ups with the track team. At that point, running had always been a nightmare for me.

I had always been behind the pack whenever we had to do physical fitness tests. There was always the mile run component. It was always 13-15 minutes of complete suffering for me. It was hell on my lungs trying to move my body around at a strong pace. It hurt like crazy on my knees. I never used long distance running as a part of my workouts because it was always so hard and painful. In that moment on the scale, none of that mattered. If running was the path to freedom, then so be it. I was accustomed to being in pain, so it didn't matter.

That day at the scale in front of GNC, I made a quick plan: No more soda, No more sweets, No more fast food, and No more fried foods. I would give myself one cheat meal per week to break those rules. I started running every day.

For the first time in the process, the wind seemed to be at my back and I was determined to capitalize.

Catharsis

The next week the scale printed out a number: 293 lbs. GO TIME!

The following week in the high 280's.

Sometimes the number would stay the same or go up slightly. I would respond by pushing myself extra hard the following week. Pure determination was surging through my veins. I didn't care about anything else. I was heavily overtraining and I was getting weaker in the weight room. It didn't matter. There was even a girl I ended up taking to the prom that year. We liked each other but I was so focused on weight loss that it didn't matter. Any acquaintances I had from school didn't matter. On the day of our graduation I didn't want to be there. We walked across the stage, I drove home, changed my clothes, and went to the gym. Nothing else mattered.

Over eight months from January to August of 2000, I worked out like a mad man. I held true to my rules about dieting. I lost 80 pounds. There was a route that I ran around my school almost daily. It was the same route we used to warm up when I was on the track team. Like I said, I hated running and in the beginning of that year, I couldn't run the route once without stopping several times to walk. By August I was running around the entire route 3 times without stopping. At the end of every run I would walk around the school track to cool off. I was always sweating heavily, but I was also crying on many days. I had been working so hard, for so long to change my body, and it was finally happening. I didn't give a damn who knew about it or if anyone acknowledged it. This was for me. I knew how hard I had been working.

Losing weight was so much more than losing weight. That process represented the removal of a yoke from around my neck. For so many years I had endured frustration with school, the teasing, the being out-shined in athletics, and the challenges of home life. I was now going off to college 80 pounds lighter and I didn't have to take shit off people anymore. I was free. Suddenly, I was reinvigorated. As grueling as the workouts were, I had found a resurgence of energy for life. The burnout I had begun my senior year with, gave way to a new hope for the future with every pound that I shed.

When I would finish up my runs on the track I would walk and relish the emotions that I had running through me. I would think about all the times I fell to the back of the class in runs on the PE test. Like I said before, it was common for females to outperform me on pull ups. Whenever we would do the pull up portion of the physical fitness test, I would usually hang for 60 seconds pulling with all my might but failing to do a single repetition. Pure embarrassment and my classmates and the teacher would let me know I should be embarrassed. That summer during cool down walks on the track I would sometimes stop and do pull ups on the soccer goal that was on the field. I would crank out 10 reps easily. It was satisfaction on a whole new level.

I would look down at my feet sometimes. I could stand straight up and look down and see my feet. I could bend straight over to tie my shoes. I couldn't do this before. I would have to sit down and work my way around my belly to tie my shoes. I had climbed Mt. Everest and on many days at the end of my cool down all I could think about was, "If I could bottle this feeling up and give it to people, I would."

I went through a total metamorphosis in that 8 month period. It was much more than my body that had changed. I had experienced a catharsis. I barely stopped to relish the fact that I wasn't in school anymore. When you have been pushing against an immovable object for 7 long years... you've dug your heels in... you've cried yourself to sleep on many nights because you feel defeated, over and over again... you get up and re-engage after being defeated, over and over again... when you get laughed at and mocked, year after year... when coaches scold you for being weak or slow... When you confront this negative energy, year after year, but you keep pushing and you keep showing up... then finally something moves... it's a feeling that I can't fully describe.

I knew that I had done something that many people struggle their whole lives to do. At 18 years old, I felt as though I had a responsibility to share what I had learned with others. I had learned some practical things about exercise and diet that were super simple: Eat less and move more. I didn't have the best balance but it really was that simple. What I didn't realize is the lesson in mental toughness

41

that I had been gaining through all those years in my K-12 education. I had been learning mental stamina, grit, and resilience without knowing it. I was developing character. This sort of commitment to a goal became my standard and that would prove to be a significant asset as I moved on to college.

PERSONAL OWNERSHIP PRINCIPLE #1:
ACTION OVER TIME

If it's worth having, it's worth fighting for...

We don't control time. We can't rewind time, fast forward it, pause it, or stop it. However, we can control our focus and how we use our energy relative to time. We can control our actions. Any meaningful goal in life will most likely take a relatively long period of time to accomplish. With significant time comes both adversity and opportunity. The key is to continue to act in the face of adversity so that we are able to reach the opportunity.

Dealing with adversity while pursuing an important goal creates a sense of struggle and it's often difficult to recognize how intense struggles are shaping us while we're in the fight. I certainly didn't know how the struggles of my childhood were transforming me while I was fighting hard to lose weight.

7 years is a long time for anyone to strive aggressively for any goal. However, as long as that goal is deeply meaningful to the individual, I say keep going! My health was, and is, important to me. To me, health and longevity is something worth having. It was my firm conviction as a child that I should fight for it, no matter what I had to

fight through, whether I ultimately achieved it or not. As time passed, conditions beyond my control shifted in my favor.

When I was losing all that weight so many years ago, I would have told you that persistence, doggedness, and determination were the keys to my success. This is partially true. What I wasn't aware of at 18 years old is the fact that my actions existed in a broader context. I never took time to conceptualize what life after K-12 education would be like. During this phase of my life my waking hours were spent at school or at home. Both situations were sources of intense stress. I had no other reference point back then, so I didn't know I was under so much pressure. It's only been in the last 5-6 years that I have been able to see that in hindsight.

Whether I graduated or not, high school was going to end and the stress associated with it would subside. That has nothing to do with my level of persistence or willingness to work hard. That's just time and the nature of K-12 public education. Both of which are beyond my control. When the stressful conditions of school went away, I suddenly had the mental clarity to change my diet. This allowed me to capitalize on the well formed habit of exercise, that I had been cultivating for 7 years... even though my exercise strategy was terrible.

What if I had let the bullying cause me to lose heart and give up on the process? What if I let the shame, disappointment, and failure steal my hope? What if I never started because I didn't have access to a gym, a personal trainer, or family members who were athletic? I wouldn't have been able to take advantage of the opportunity because I wouldn't have been in the process.

Over 7 years... The repetition of getting up early in the morning during the summertime, day after day, to put myself through brutal workouts. The repetition of writing down my workouts on yellow legal pads for 7 years trying different routines and reviewing numbers trying to scrutinize why I wasn't seeing any real change. The repetition of trying to eat in a healthier way and failing miserably, only to ask myself, "Why can't I stop eating so much sugar and junk food?" The repetition of facing my peers at school, having them call me fat and ugly, crying myself to sleep, and using that pain as a source of energy to workout the next day... There is a difference between having knowledge and embodying that knowledge. By engaging with the struggle to exercise consistently and eat a healthy diet, I embodied these habits. Lots of people know they should exercise regularly and eat a quality diet, but so few people do it because they give up on the process when life presents challenges to it. Or worse, they never get started because they're waiting on more information, or more resources, or more ideal life circumstances. If you never engage the process, how do you know what ideal circumstances look like?

In a way, adversity is an opportunity. Adversity helped to solidify a mindset, *'When something is important to you, you fight for it no matter what!'* In this sense, mindset towards a meaningful goal is more important than strategy to achieve the goal. The adversity of my childhood gave me an opportunity to fortify my mindset. This mindset helped me stay in the process long enough to reach a point of strategic advantage. In this example I'm talking about exercise and diet but you can extrapolate this principle to any significant goal. The more time you spend on it, the more adversity you are likely to face in pursuing it. If you engage with adversity, it will make your mind stronger and this will keep you in the process longer. The longer you're in the process, the more likely you are to experience a window of opportunity. Of course, there are never guarantees that you will reach your goals but, *if it's worth having, it's worth fighting for.*

PART II - STORY

A Sincere Compliment

Somewhere between 70-80 lbs... that's how much weight I lost before heading off to college at The University of Houston (UH) in August 2000. It was exciting. I was even beginning to get compliments from women. Surreal. Going to my Senior Prom had been a miracle in my head. It was the first date I had ever been on and we had a good time. Who knew I was a fun date?

However, my perception of myself wouldn't really allow me to get comfortable with being attractive to women. It was me against the world and women being interested in me just didn't fit with the story:

'She just came to the prom to show pity on me...'

'She's flirting with me because she wants to take advantage of me or make a joke out of me in some way...'

These are the thoughts that would go through my head. I didn't see any problem with it because this is where I had been living in my mind for years. I was the persecuted hero in my own narrative even though the compliments and flirting were direct evidence to the contrary. I held tight to my story. After all, my story helped me win a seven year battle to lose weight. There had to be some value in it.

Back to Reality

I was leaving Birmingham behind. I would come home to visit my parents, but that would be it. All the people I went to school with and all the painful memories were about to be erased from my mind. Houston was going to be a new start. A place where I was no longer timid. A place where people respected me. A place where I would be studying something I was naturally interested in. Growing up, I had spent lots of time by myself, tinkering with electronics trying to figure out how they worked. I would take old radios and break them down only to get to the circuit board with all of its different components and say to myself, "One day I have to figure out how this works." I was going to major in Electrical Engineering and build things that improved people's lives. That was the goal.

I even thought that maybe one day I could combine my interest in electronics with my passion for exercise and health. Maybe I would Minor in Kinesiology. UH had a good Exercise Science Department. Also, I wanted to try out for UH's baseball team. I had big plans. College was going to be liberating. People had talked about college being one of the best times in a person's life and after years of struggling with different issues I was ready for some fun.

I had earned partial academic scholarships from the Cullen College of Engineering at the UH Main Campus. To keep my scholarships I had to take a full-time course load and maintain a minimum 3.0 grade point average (GPA) in all of my engineering classes. A full-time course load was considered 12 hours but the way the Electrical Engineering Degree Plan was laid out, the first semesters involved at least 15 hours. It was 15 hours assuming that you would be starting your mathematics course work in Calculus. The degree plan would take a total of 5 years if you took summers off and stayed at about 15 hours a semester.

Right from the start, the task was sobering. There was a math placement test I had to take as an Engineering Major. Almost all the other students I started with placed into Calculus as the degree plan laid out. I didn't qualify to start in Calculus. I began in Pre- Calculus. From the beginning, I was behind in a degree program that already took 5 years to complete if you started at the right place. That first semester of school I was enrolled in 16 credit hours. I would be enrolled in 17 credit hours in the Spring semester. Starting that Fall Semester, the workload hit me hard. I was placed as a roommate with a couple of other freshmen. Sean was majoring in Psychology and Lane was majoring in Communications. Lane had a close friend, James, who I would also become close to. He was majoring in Business. They were all enrolled in 12 hour course loads.

It became very clear, very quickly, that I was going to have to work hard. Really hard. From the start, I was staying up all night to understand homework assignments, finish papers, or cram for tests. I was trying to have some kind of social life, but it was nothing compared to what my friends were doing. They weren't partying like crazy but they seemed to have a much more relaxed pace and lower level of intensity with their studies than I had with mine. It wasn't just the difference in majors either. Lane had a fairly challenging home life. I would argue more so than mine but he didn't seem to have the same sense of urgency about academic success as I did. Another thing I noticed was the fact that other people seemed to be more confident in their abilities than I was. I was confident in my work ethic but not in my natural intelligence. Academically, I knew I had to put in work to do well.

On top of academics and some measure of social interaction, I was still working out hard. I still had weight to lose. Also, that first year would see me deal with a financial curveball. My stepfather got laid off of work. The original financial aid application that I turned in, reflected a family income that was much higher than reality. The first two semesters of college I spent many hours in the financial aid office working on proving my parents' new, lower income level. This would get me more financial aid as I was threatened with being dropped from my courses both semesters of my freshman year, for failure to pay tuition. I didn't have the money to pay and, true to my mother's warning when I was young, my parents didn't have it either.

My family in Houston was another challenge that I hadn't foreseen coming down the road. In particular, my older sister was difficult. She was 9 years older than me and growing up in Houston, I had always looked up to her. She was my hero. She was smart and it seemed like she was relatively popular at school because she brought friends to the apartment sometimes. In my head, she was sort of a rock star but when I got to college her behavior didn't quite match the idea I had of her. She and other family members would ask to borrow money from me which they never returned. I found myself spending time helping them with their lives, much more often than them helping me with mine. It was a hard reality to accept because I held my sister and other family members in high esteem. I didn't want to see them as being irresponsible or taking advantage of me, but in hindsight, that's what was happening.

College had been built up in my head to be this great time in life of creating lifelong friends through common studies and memorable social interactions. This was not going to be my reality. Obstacles besieged my college experience immediately and it was clear that a minor in exercise science may not happen and tryouts for baseball may not happen. I barely had time for a little bit of social life. In response to these challenges, I did what I knew best: I put my head down and grinded.

False Summit

For the first time in my life, I had close friends. It was a good thing, but it also presented new problems. Growing up, I didn't hang out with other kids outside of school. In the summertime, I was always alone. I didn't go to birthday parties or any sort of social functions when I was in Birmingham. Looking back, I can remember my mother asking questions about this lack of social interaction because it concerned her. But it was normal to me. Was I being bullied? Yes, but, outside of school, I was in my own world and I wasn't going to invite anyone into it if I didn't have to. In grade school, life was better alone. Of course, this means I wasn't developing social skills and that's a problem in new relationships.

One of the big challenges I had in college, initially, was learning how to take a joke and learning how to take constructive criticism. Men joke with each other. Especially young men. However, in my world, joking had never really been joking. I had always been the butt of the joke and other people were laughing at me, not with me. I had made a promise to myself that this would not be the case in my new life in college. There were many times where I would snap at people for no reason. James commented that I was often short on the phone with my parents. I was frustrated with them as well. I felt as though I had taken lots of criticism from my mother when I lived at home. I was an adult. If I wanted to be mean to her, I was going to be mean to her. James was particularly patient in pointing out some of the flaws in my communication style. He came to me and said, "I'm telling you this because I care about you, but people think your behavior is strange sometimes... You snap at small things or little jokes people make, just having fun with you..."

At first, I was defensive and I didn't want to hear it. In my head I had always been the lone persecuted hero and, up until college, there had been nothing in my surroundings to challenge that narrative. This time was the real beginning of self-examination and deep introspection for me. It wasn't purely about pleasing people. I desperately wanted to be understood. I could identify why certain things made me snap. They reminded me of my childhood that was still painfully fresh in my mind. The idea that I could simply move away from those traumatic experiences was beginning to fall apart.

I wanted friendships, I wanted people to understand me, and I knew that the first step was the admission that I had a problem. My picture of myself as the triumphant hero overcoming all odds, who was perfect and virtuous, was false. I had some work to do. Much more work than I fully understood at the time. It was a hard thing to accept. I was the one who had been treated so poorly by other people for no reason, for so long. I never received one apology from anyone, for anything that was said about me or done to me. Why did I have to work on myself? Why couldn't I just be mad? Why did I have to apologize for my errors when others never apologized for theirs? Never-the-less, I wanted to have friends, so I did the only thing that seemed logical. I asked people to forgive me for my outbursts and I worked to control my reactions to the ups and downs of friendships. It was a humbling time.

When I reflect upon this particular time in my life, I see how much I was holding on to my own pain. I think we often feel that our freedom from an emotional burden is tied to someone else's admission of guilt. I think this sets us up to live in a perpetual state of holding grievances against someone or something. In this case I was mad at all my classmates and my family for how difficult my childhood had been. This was limiting my ability to connect with others. My own personal experience of trauma and grief had become supreme and uniquely hurtful. More so than the experiences of others. Fortunately, I was able to look at myself in this situation because I was accustomed to facing reality and taking personal responsibility for that reality.

I realized that people had to feel safe with me before they were willing to try to understand me. I had to have the humility to recognize that my narrative was incomplete at best, and utterly wrong at worst. Everyone is not my enemy or why would I want friends? If I was perfectly virtuous, why was I seeking to hurt my mother's feelings at times?

Also, I was probably on edge because I was stressed out like crazy. I was having issues with family, financial struggles, and massive academic challenges. My own social awkwardness was a huge issue. When I first showed up to UH I only had the clothes that I had worn during my senior year in high school. But I had been 305 lbs during my senior year in high school. I had lost 80 lbs at this point, so all my clothes hung off of me. I remember not having decent shoes initially. I had worn out my shoes with all the heavy workouts I was doing. So I wore sandals a lot. Often, I wore those sandals with royal blue socks that I had from playing baseball in high school. It was not a fashionable look to say the least. It made me self conscious among other things. I just wasn't comfortable in my own skin.

When you're hiking up an incline in the woods, you may look ahead and see what looks like the top. Then you get there and realize there's another long incline in front of you. That's a false summit. Depending on how tired you are, it can be deflating. This is how I felt in my freshman year of college. I had done all that work to lose weight. I had reached the summit, or so I thought. I wasn't deflated, but it was all incredibly sobering.

Electromagnetic Waves

I could spend many pages and words telling you about various academic challenges I had in college. To sum it up, engineering is really hard and I'm not the smartest person in the world. The advantage that I had academically was the fact that I was accustomed to working hard on a problem for a long time. I was also accustomed to working from a deficit. One class in particular highlights my use of both of those tools: Introduction to Electromagnetic Wave Theory.

Yes. A mouthful. And, Yes. It was as hard as it sounds. I took this class in the fall semester of my third year in college. It was a class that was notorious for weeding people out of the Electrical Engineering Program. I came close to being a casualty myself.

The information was complicated and I had to spend long nights grinding my mental gears in the library, just to comprehend the homework. At this point in my college experience it was common to spend weekends studying all day. One of the things that I thought was a little sadistic on the part of the Engineering College is the fact that exams were often scheduled for Saturday Mornings. So you would go through a week of crushing yourself studying and doing homework, just to get to Friday night and watch all your non-engineering friends go off and start a fun weekend while your work was just beginning. I'm sure they had their reason for the way they scheduled things but it was brutal. In grade school it never dawned on me that such a thing would be possible. The weekend was the weekend and when Friday came you were done, right? Nope. There were many exams I took on a Friday. I would finish and go get something to eat and then head right back to the library. The library often closed before I was done studying. This meant heading over to the Engineering Building where people often stayed all night studying. I was one of those people.

The first exam in Electromagnetics was a large percentage of our final grade. I had another exam on the same day in another class that was also a weed-out class, Circuit Analysis. I stayed up all night on Friday night studying. I came into both exams exhausted. Electromagnetics was first. It was hard. Afterwards we all gathered and talked about the exam questions and how we felt about our answers. I realized quickly that I made some gross errors on most of the exam questions. I took the Circuits exam and did fine, but I made a 38/100 on the Electromagnetics Exam. The exam was worth somewhere between 30-40% of our overall grade. When I went to pick up my exam from the professor, he looked at me with sincere concern and recommended that I drop the course. It was still early enough in the semester that the grade wouldn't count against my GPA.

In hindsight, I knew he meant well in his recommendation that I drop. However, I didn't take it that way. In my mind he was saying that I wasn't smart enough to handle this course. He was saying that I didn't have what it takes. He was calling me fat, slow, and stupid. Sometimes emotional triggers work against you and sometimes they work for you. In response to his recommendation, I did what I knew best: I put my head down and grinded.

Work Work

Whether it was because I just didn't comprehend the information, or I was too sleepy to make good decisions, or just made a bunch of silly errors, in looking at the exam I realized that I had executed a poor understanding of the basic theories we had learned in class. I was determined to stay in this class and pass it. I took all of our homework assignments and went back to the beginning. I began working through the homework problems and going back through the textbook from the beginning. This meant ramping up my study time. Friday, Saturday, and Sundays became days for review and mastering the basic concepts of the class. The other days of the week were for my other scheduled classes. I went to office hours with the professor and his teaching assistants. I got help from classmates. I worked hard to deepen my understanding and after a few weeks I began to feel very confident in my grasp of the material.

We took the second exam and then the final exam. I made scores of 80% and 96% respectively. We had one final project on which I scored a 95%. My efforts would bring my overall grade up from failing, to a B+. We had to go and pick up our final projects from the professor in order to get our grades. He did that so he could review our overall grades with us. When he handed me my project and looked over my final scores for the semester, he had a sort of shocked look on his face. I remember him saying, "Wow! You had to come back from a long way! Good Work!" I've never forgotten that look on his face. It was satisfying. I could tell that he couldn't remember recommending that I drop the class. To be fair to him, there were lots of students enrolled in the class. Lots of faces to remember. And, in hindsight, I know he was only making the recommendation he thought was best for me. Lots of people failed that class and had to retake it. For many people, that class became the course that made them choose another major.

Seeing that look on my professor's face, reminded me of the looks I would get from old classmates while home in Birmingham on winter break. I have to admit, it's an intoxicating feeling to inspire that 'wow' factor in people. Whether I was born with it or my experiences as a kid put it in me, I am competitive with almost everything I do. I'm coming for you. Whether my story about you being my enemy is true or false, I'll make you my enemy for as long as I need to, to win. That's the power of our stories.

Electromagnetics was one course among many where I had to dig deep and find a way to win. All night study sessions and very little in the way of relaxation marked my college experience. Whenever we had breaks for Thanksgiving and Spring Break, I stayed in the dorms studying because it was quiet and I always had work to catch up on. Using those breaks meant I could try to get ahead. It was a brutal pace to keep for five years. As I hit my 4th and 5th years in college, my brain and body were becoming less capable of maintaining that same intensity of effort. I couldn't sustain that pace forever and I never took the time to ask myself whether I was happy with being an Engineer. Maybe because I was trying to find that happiness elsewhere...

Searching for Satisfaction

With all the academic work taking up so much of my bandwidth, I still had a dream. I still felt that if I could get onto a baseball team, I had the potential to do well. If I could get access to the right coaching, I felt my ability to grind and solve problems could take me a good distance in baseball. I ended up trying out for UH's baseball team twice while I was in college. It was a horrible showing both times. I just couldn't find the time nor the energy to really prepare myself for the process. When I look back on it, I really think what I was trying to do was find something fun. Find something enjoyable to do. Find something other than studying and part-time work. But that was also combined with a deep need to prove myself to people, to show people that I mattered. To show the young women that weren't giving me the time of day that I was a decent guy. To show the coaches and teammates that I had in highschool that they should have given me more of a chance. I was looking for satisfaction and validation.

My interaction with women in college was challenging. I was learning how to approach women for the first time and it often took me weeks to build up the courage to say something to a young lady. Once I did say something, it was often accompanied by jitters and sweating. I got the run-around pretty good one time from a girl that I liked a lot. Dealing with the fallout was extremely painful. I was growing up and learning that romance was complicated. Looking back, I can recognize that there were young women who were interested in me. However, again, my narrative about myself just wouldn't let me embrace that. I struggled with rejection and for a long time I let those denials cause me to think that something was wrong with me. *'Maybe I am still the fat disgusting kid I was in highschool... Maybe I am doomed to be alone...'* In reality, with romantic interest, you win some and you lose some. Women will tell a man *'no'* for a litany of reasons, even when you're a solid dude. That's life and it's okay.

Me being who I am, I used the rejection as drive and motivation to get up and continue to workout, continue to attack my classes, and continue to try to improve my level of self confidence. It was around this time in college that I began thinking about my sources of validation and the need to validate myself. It would take time to get good at this but losing out on baseball and women made me look within and it was a good revelation.

After the last baseball tryout in college I went back to my dorm room and I layed on the floor. I cried. I reminisced about crying in front of my teammates in the dugout in highschool. The persistent disappointment was heartbreaking. I felt like all I had to look forward to was school work and that was becoming more and more miserable. I will always enjoy a challenge but at some point you want to be interested in the challenge you are engaged with. You want to feel like you are doing something that's meaningful to you. I never even looked at what it would take to minor in Exercise Science. The academic workload of engineering had sucked all the air out of my lunges. I was walking away from baseball disappointed with the result but I was at total peace with my level of effort. It was a little strange at the time, but I could live with the failure because I knew I had done all I could with what I had. I was ready to let go. It was a similar feeling to failing out of the Gifted and Talented Program back when I was in elementary school. Baseball was the same lesson, though disappointing, failure is tolerable in light of giving my best effort.

Internship

My first internship came with one of the major American Car Manufacturers in Detroit, MI. Ford Motor Company. After my third year in college I went up to Michigan for the summer to intern. I was excited to get real world experience as opposed to the theoretical learning I had been doing in class. I was also motivated to prove myself and show that I belonged. Despite a lot of effort, getting an internship had been out of reach the first two summers I was in college. It was something that was crucial to getting a job offer after graduation. I was motivated to show the engineers in Michigan I was a hard worker and I did just that. For three months in the Summer of 2003, I did every project I could stick my hand in and I worked after the regular work day when asked. Again, I never asked myself whether or not I enjoyed the work.

The other big factor in being so motivated to get the internship was the fact that I was always broke. Financially, I was always barely surviving. I knew other engineers that worked almost full time and went to school full time. I couldn't see how they did it. I spent so much time studying that even 15 hours a week at my campus job was a lot. Studying outside of class time was a fulltime job plus overtime for me. Of course, I also made it a point to workout at least 3x/week and I tried to cook my own food when I could. I was still very dedicated to staying in good physical shape and, perhaps, if I were willing to gain the 'freshman 15' as it's called, I would have had more time to work. Nevertheless, being broke blinded me from paying attention to the overall internship experience during that first summer. I wasn't asking myself questions about interest and job satisfaction. How was I going to feel about engineering 10 years in? These things didn't cross my mind. I was there to put my head down, make money, and impress my coworkers. I got invited back the next summer after my fourth year in college.

Originally, my plan was to get my undergrad degree and go to graduate school. At the time, Ford had a program that paid for graduate school if you came and worked for them afterwards. However, after my fourth year in school, I began to question that plan. A graduate degree and maybe a PhD at some point, was always the plan when I was growing up. The higher the education, the higher the prestige, and the more success I would enjoy in life. That had been the idea I had lodged in my head. The problem was the fact that I was starting to crash. Whereas in previous years I was able to stay up all night, multiple nights in a row studying, in my second to last year of undergrad, I could barely make it past 11 pm. Even when I did stay up, my concentration was weak at best. I got through my 4th year, but it was a blur. Truth be told, the whole of college was a blur.

When I went for the second summer internship, I noticed things I hadn't noticed the first time. I was at a desk both summers but in the second summer it was bothering me in a way that I hadn't noticed before. Even my part-time job during the school year involved deskwork that I didn't like, but it was part time. I realized that staring at the computer screen all day was a major source of frustration. I started to complain a bit about the boredom and one of my coworkers snapped at me. I realized something was changing. I was doing baseball workouts during the week after work. I was getting up before work to do strength and conditioning. I was motivated for those things, but not the internship itself.

While in Michigan that second summer I told my mother over the phone that the original plan of graduate school was over with. I was tired. I was beginning to wonder if Engineering was the right choice. I had one year left. I was definitely going to finish. My hope was that if I just took some time off from school and poured more into my other interests, then maybe the drive to go to graduate school would return. When my fifth and final fall semester came around after the second internship, I continued to work out in efforts to try out for the baseball team. As had been the pattern, quickly, my academic work became so overwhelming that the workouts suffered. By the time the tryout came, I was nowhere near as good as I had been over the summer. I think this is another reason why it hurt so bad. If I could just get the consistent time and repetition, I knew I could be good but engineering always took priority. That would have been fine if I were passionate about engineering above all else. However, in reality, I was beginning to realize that I didn't give a damn about engineering.

What I really wanted to do was be involved in athletics and help other people get in better physical shape. These were my passions but I had gotten so fixated on *'being successful'* that had never given those passions an opportunity to breathe. Also, I think that I am a glutton for punishment. I thrive off of challenges and engineering gave me just that. I hadn't ever thought about whether I enjoyed it or not. I had this idea that once I was working and making money, I would be happy and the drudgery would be worth it.

I also had my family's words in my ear. My ideas about success were heavily influenced by home life. My sister who was 9 years older, had moved from one college major to another for a while. She would be enrolled one semester and take the next off. I can't remember how I interpreted that. She was still my hero and a major influence in me choosing to attend the University of Houston. My family saw her approach to college as flaky and indecisive. I heard about it a lot. *'Your sister isn't doing this or that...'* I thought of her as someone who could do no wrong but they thought of her as someone doing everything wrong. The reality was much more complicated.

If I changed majors, would I now be seen as being flaky or indecisive? Academics was the one thing I consistently got praise for, and I didn't want to lose that. The desire for validation was definitely a major influence in my continued pursuit of engineering despite a deep interest in other professions and a lack of real interest in engineering.

What is Success?

If I could just get a good job after graduation, I would be happy. I would be making good money and that would clearly mean I had become successful. That was the goal. The idea of money being correlated to success in life was enhanced greatly during my time in college. I didn't have a car the first couple years I was at UH and when I did get a car it was a beater that I paid $900 for. A 1991 Plymouth Acclaim. Talk about your grandma's car. The next car I got was after that first internship. A 1991 Acura Legend. It was much nicer, but Houston has a car culture and I was at the bottom of the hierarchy.

Whether it's tricked out old school Chevy's, souped up Tuner Cars similar to those in the *Fast and Furious* movies, or European Sedans that cost way more than any college student should be able to afford, there were nice cars everywhere. When you are driving a rolling sauna to work every day in the summer because your air conditioner doesn't work, and you're surrounded by all these beautiful cars, you can't help but think, *'One day that'll be me...'* Especially when you're 20 years old and you want to fit in and be cool because you've never fit in and you've never been cool.

Growing up, I envied the kids whose families drove nice cars. I've always been intrigued by the idea of the automobile and the freedom that comes with owning your own car has always been alluring. My first car was a 1987 Ford Tempo that my parents gave me in my junior year of high school (1999). I remember getting ready to go to my high school senior prom. Again, given the context, this seemed miraculous on many levels. I had never been to any kind of school dance up until that point and I had never been on a date either. It was a lot of pressure for someone who had struggled socially throughout school.

In a conversation with one of my teammates from baseball, I was asked what kind of car I would drive to the prom. I replied sheepishly, "My Ford Tempo..." He laughed. I had to do something. I had suffered enough embarrassment from being a fat kid, I wasn't about to be laughed at, at the prom. I begged my parents to rent me a car for the night. They agreed. *'One day, I gotta have a better car...'*, I'd think to myself.

As I said, Houston has a car culture and my auto-envy started at a young age. Over the years moving into college, quietly and subconsciously, I had attached much of my identity to my vehicle status. I had lost weight but I still wasn't cool. I still wasn't good enough. I was still seeking external validation. I didn't know it. I was unaware of myself. I was too distracted by school and wanting to fit in. When I bought that Plymouth Acclaim I was grateful but in my mind I said, "I have to have a better car." Notice the, *'have to'*.

I drove my Plymouth for about 9-10 months until it died just after finishing my junior year of college. That summer I headed to Michigan to do my first internship with Ford Motor Company. I went to Michigan with no car. Of course, in Motor City, working for one of the Big Three, my auto-envy was on fire. One of my work mentors found out I didn't have a car and he let me use his 2003 S-Type Jaguar for one week and later on he let me use his 2003 Ford Explorer for a week. I was like, *'Dang! One day, I gotta have a better car!'* The car envy was growing rapidly at the time.

During my 4th year of college, I finally had enough money to buy a decent car (the 1991 Acura Legend I mentioned earlier). It was in decent shape and I considered it somewhat of a classic. Of course, the AC didn't work. In Houston, of all places. Story of my life. Eventually, before going off to Ford for my second internship, I got the AC fixed. I was good for about 1 week and then one day while driving on the interstate, something bounced off the ground and hit the car under the engine. A loud crack was immediately followed by a loud hissing sound. That hissing was the sound of the freon leaking out of the AC system I had just gotten repaired a week earlier. All I could do was laugh. It was amazing! Luckily for me I was heading off to Michigan for my second summer in a row and I didn't need AC but you've got to love the irony. I drove that car for the remainder of my time in college and eventually got the AC repaired... again.

There's a reason I'm walking you through my personal vehicle history. This car-envy played a pivotal role in a decision I made after college that proved to have a significant impact on my life. It's very hard to be aware of how our material cravings can override not only our sensibilities in terms of spending habits, but they can also threaten our ability to have options in life. I had done all this academic work and put all this sweat equity into my body, but I hadn't really challenged myself to sit and think about what a successful and fulfilled life was, to me. In college I saw how well people dressed and the nice cars that people drove and that seemed like something that would make me feel better about myself. Our image of self is so underdeveloped at this time in life (early 20's) yet we're inundated by images and ideas of what we should and shouldn't be doing. No one was really asking me to think deeply about what I wanted. It's fair to say that most people at this age, don't know, that they don't know what they want for their futures.

'Travis, What excites you? What are you interested in?'

If I was asking these questions, I wasn't doing anything of consequence with the answers. There were many days I thought about changing my major from engineering to exercise science. I was much more interested in the latter. But exercise science just didn't fit the success model.

By this time in my life I had well formed archetypes of success that already existed in the broader consciousness of society and I was simply adopting them: A good paying job, A nice car, A house, A Wife and Children, Nice Clothes, Vacations, 401K etc. My 4th year in college I began thinking about what it might be like to actually own my own gym and help people get in shape. I know I said I was done with baseball but not quite. I still had dreams of being a baseball player and I would eventually go to an open tryout for the Houston Astros after college. Another, very unsuccessful attempt. Owning a gym was something that was more reasonable of a goal in one way but much more intimidating in other ways.

I loved being physical and working to improve my skill in a sport. It was challenging and fun. That's why baseball made sense in one way. Obviously, making money doing it was a long shot. Making a liveable income by owning my own business was much more of a possibility. Especially in light of my personal experience. However, I had no examples of business owners in my life. When I brought up the idea, people reacted to it as a distant second to engineering. I also had this false belief that business owners had to be extroverts and have some hidden knowledge that I didn't have access to. I was an engineer and conditioned myself to look for a job in order to have an income. Owning my own profitable business seemed like a dream that was even further away than professional baseball. The goal of helping other people lose weight and improve their lives was always in the back of my head, but having a business felt impossible. I didn't feel like I had the skills to make it work.

Finishing College

There isn't a whole lot to say about my time in college. It was a grind. Work, Work, and more Work. I got two job offers in my senior year. One from Ford Motor in Detroit and another from Shell Oil in New Orleans. I had decided that I was no longer willing to leave Houston. I had spent 5 years crushing myself and I wanted to be able to spend time with the friends I had made in college. I turned down the offer from Ford but I knew Shell had offices in Houston. I asked if I could be reassigned and they did it. If not, the plan was to just keep looking for local jobs. I had fallen across the finish line to graduate. I wasn't excited about starting my new job. I was relieved that college was over. I was exhausted. More specifically, I think I was tired of being miserable. At that point, my whole life had been about pushing through some massive obstacle. There was so much disappointment and very little in the way of joy.

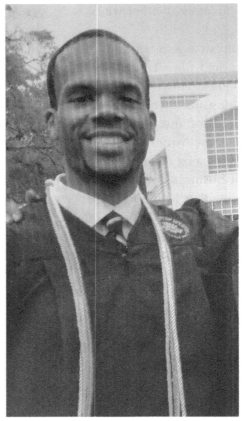

(The Day I graduated from UH. May 13, 2005)

I hated school. From elementary school all the way through college, I hated the entire thing. I worked hard at it because I wanted to be successful and this is what successful people did, right? There were many things I had assumed about engineering. I thought that I would be doing cool little robotics projects all through my degree track. I did one the entire time. One year during winter break, I was at the halfway point in my degree. My stepfather asked me a question, "So can you work on the wiring in the house now?" After all, I was an Electrical Engineer. I was ashamed to admit that I had very little in the way of practical skills. I thought those skills would come eventually, but they never did. Just lots of theory. The burnout I was beginning to feel at the end of college was real. I began to talk of being frustrated with engineering and, right away, I had people begin telling me how I should be grateful that I had a job offer. Today I realize that I had no balance. It's hard to be grateful for certain things when there is very little sense of purpose, joy, or happiness in your life. I had chosen a path of almost constant drudgery and I was beginning to break down. Add to that, the hard road that life had been before college, and it's easy to see a mounting frustration and disillusionment happening in my mind. Something had to give.

Commuting

Shell gave me a job at its West Houston location. My first day of work was in August, about 3 months after graduation. My starting salary in 2005 was $59,000 per year, plus performance bonuses. 18 years later, I still think that's an incredible starting salary for anyone fresh out of college. I was hoping that the money and relief from the constant churn of academics would be a reprieve. I was hoping for more time with friends and maybe even romance. I was hoping to be interested in the work. I still remember walking up to the building on the first day and saying aloud to myself, "I'm going to hate this."

One of the first errors I made was getting a relatively nice apartment with my good friend, James. At this point, we were like brothers. The error wasn't in living with him, it was in the choice of location. We were living close to the center of the city in an apartment that was far more expensive than what we needed. I wasn't thinking in terms of transitioning away from engineering. I was listening to other people tell me how grateful I should be. I had achieved success and everyone was so proud of me, so I have to enjoy it, right?

The commute from the center of the city to my office in West Houston took an hour on most morningings and up to 2 hours on the return home in the afternoon. I worked in what was known as The Energy Corridor. There are offices for all the major oil and gas companies along the stretch of road known as Dairy Ashford. If I could go back, I would have put myself on an 18 month timeline. I would have lived within a 15-20 minute walk from work, in a studio apartment. I would have bought a mattress to sleep on and no other furniture. I would have budgeted hard. I only had $22,000 in student loans. I brought home about $48,000 after taxes for the 11 months that I worked at Shell. Today, I know that I can live comfortably on $1600/month. If you do the math, I pay off my student loans in 11 months while still having $763/month for savings. I can live comfortably on $1600/month in 2023 numbers. In 2005, I would have been set.

With that plan, I would have been able to walk away from engineering with no issues. However, I wasn't willing to admit to myself that I was miserable. I didn't have the courage to stand up to people who had no idea what I was going through internally. I wanted to please other people more than myself. Most of my closest friends and family members wouldn't hear of it when I expressed frustration with my situation. It was all about the money and security. I understand it now but it was intensely frustrating at the time. Just like when I was a kid, I stuffed the frustration down and tried to soldier on.

But I was running out of gas.

Car Trouble

Soon after starting my new job, I came out to my car one morning and it wouldn't start up. After an hour of fiddling around, I finally got it started. I can remember saying to myself that morning, "I deserve a new car!" I still had car-envy but now I had some significant money coming into my bank account. Combined with the apprehension I felt towards the job itself, it was a recipe for a bad decision.

The 2005 Atlantic Hurricane Season was record breaking. 3 weeks after Hurricane Katrina had displaced so many people from Louisiana into Texas, Hurricane Rita was forcing everyone to evacuate Houston. Many people drove towards Dallas. The freeways were like parking lots from all the traffic. I chose to drive east, home to Birmingham. It was towards where the hurricane would land but I calculated that we had enough time to get through the hot zone before the storm hit. The freeway would be wide open because everyone else was going the opposite direction. During the trip, my power steering started to fail in my Acura Legend. Obviously, this was not what we needed while running away from a hurricane and in the wrong direction. My best friend James, my older sister, and my 3 year old nephew were riding with me. My sister could be incredibly challenging at times. She was insistent about stopping at a Walmart to get some clothes for the baby. I was adamant that she could do that when we got to Birmingham because the car was having trouble and... we were running from a HURRICANE!

The combination of the hurricane, the car problems, and arguing with my sister, had me on edge. When we got to Birmingham, I took the car to get looked at. It needed some significant work. I had just started working as an engineer and I didn't quite have the money to pay for it. I was tired of the lack of reliability in the cars I owned. I was frustrated at the fact that I had spent so much time working hard and sacrificing in school, and I couldn't rely on my car to evacuate me and people I loved from a potential disaster area. "Screw it! I'm getting a new car!" The storm passed and when I got back to Houston, I began looking. Two weeks later, I was driving a 2005 Subaru Legacy with a 5 year, $28,000 loan.

When I got the new car, I went from $22,000 in debt from student loans to $50,000 dollars of debt, in the span of a few hours (the time it took to complete the loan paperwork). I knew when I started working as an engineer that I probably wasn't going to like it but I had no idea how bad it would eventually get. When I bought the car I didn't think about the fact that the financial commitment equated to opportunity costs. About 3 months after I financed the car, I began to realize that I was driving the very thing that was forcing me to keep the job. As I became more depressed about the job, I began to resent the car more and more. The car meant that I didn't have freedom of movement. Ironically, the thing that represented freedom when I was a kid was now an anchor around my neck, pinning me to a situation I didn't want to be in. As I became more and more frustrated with the long commute to an office job that I hated, my anger transformed into darkness. It's a place that I never want to go again.

A Good Job

The car envy combined with an ever increasing depression caused me to make a huge strategic error in my spending. I wanted the car because I thought it would make me feel better about my situation. Cars equated to status. If I could just get this brand new car, then I would have more status and be happy. The former might have been true in some people's eyes but the latter wasn't true at all. There were people who encouraged me to get a used car because I would save money doing so. In hindsight, that's not the advice I needed. I needed someone to acknowledge that I was miserable and had been that way for my entire life. My whole life had been pure will and determination to get through one miserable situation after another. There was hardly any room for the things I enjoyed.

Had someone said to me, *'Travis, tell me how much debt you're in. How much money do you need to live without working for a year?'* I would have asked, *'Why?!'* They would have said, *'You need to get out of debt so that no one owns your time. You need to have cash in the bank so you can pay your bills while you go and experiment with some things you want to do. Some of those experiments may involve volunteer work. You need some room to play. Forget about a car! What's it going to take to get your freedom because that's what you want right now!'*

Had somebody framed the car in that context, my ears might have been open but who can say for certain. I wasn't thinking long term. Mentally and emotionally, I was shutting down and trying to ease the pain through self medicating with the car and, eventually, with food.

I was just barely getting through each day. Once hurricane season passed, things began to settle into more of a rhythm. I began traveling to South Texas every other week. McAllen, Texas is the town I would fly into. While in Houston I would go into work and try to look at the diagrams of the piping and gas systems we had in South Texas. I would get on the internet and try to learn how all of these things worked. I had an office to myself. I struggled to concentrate. Fairly quickly, there started to be talk of having me move to South Texas. That was a trajectory that all new engineers took. If I had gone to New Orleans as originally planned, my role would have taken me to a two weeks on, two weeks off, offshore oil rig job. That would have been horrible. I didn't want to move and I wasn't going to move.

It wasn't about having anything against McAllen or New Orleans. My whole life had been this marathon of brute force. Gutting my way through difficult frustrating situations that often left me depleted or filled with anger (with the exception of weight loss and athletics). I was running on empty and nothing looked attractive about this career. I wanted to stay in Houston and explore the city I had been living in for the 5 previous years, but never had the time, energy, or money to do so. I wanted to spend time with my friends and family. I wanted to enjoy life more. Instead, I was commuting at least 2 hours per day in a car I should never have bought, to go sit in an office studying things that I could care less about. But there was pressure. Parents thought I should be happy. I was a first generation college student. I'm black. I was an engineer at a big company. I had a couple of black coworkers at the time who had been doing work to get more minority representation in engineering. For them, it was a win that I was there.

I was supposed to be happy, whether I gave a damn about the job or not. My parents were born in the 50's in the deep south. For me to reach that type of career was something that they had seen denied black people for years. My older black coworkers felt the same way. This was a story of overcoming and success in their minds. I should be grateful. I wasn't and this was hard for me because whenever I expressed discontent, people corrected me, *'You should be grateful for that job!'* Lots of people projected their ideas about success and no one really concerned themselves with how I felt... to include me. I did my best to try and be grateful. After all, I was making good money and I had a nice car. I should be satisfied, right?

Then, in October, I met a young woman...

An Invite to Church

In October, I had a close female friend from college who was having a birthday party. She had a friend who I had met once before. This friend was also at the party and we sat next to one another at the dinner table. Her name was Karissa. We were locked in conversation the whole night. She was intriguing. She had just returned from being out of the country where she had done a mission's trip with her church. She was also a dancer and was part of a local dance production there in Houston. That night I saw in Karissa's eyes the spark of someone doing things that they loved. It was extremely attractive. I confessed to her that I was unhappy as an engineer. I told her how amazing I thought it was that she was following her heart.

At some point during the conversation we got on the topic of health. She said she had been working with a group of ladies from her church. Being a dancer and having been thin her whole life, she was having trouble connecting with the ladies around their struggles with weight loss. Of course, this was something that I had personal experience in. I told her some of my journey and she asked me if I would be willing to come to her Saturday class and speak with the women about my journey. I did and it was a satisfying experience to give some encouragement to a group of people trying to do the same thing I had done. I probably said something like, *'You gotta believe and be willing to work hard everyday...'* Today this makes me laugh. It's still a true statement but I've learned so much more about the layers of psychological and practical barriers that one has to work through in order to make any significant change in life. Especially losing weight. Still, it was a good moment. After the class I went and got lunch with Karissa. We had something going on and I kept coming to those Saturday classes.

Eventually, she invited me to come to the service that the church had on Sundays. I believed in God but organized religion had never been part of my life. The church had always been this nebulous institution. I felt awkward any time I found myself in a church. But for Karissa, I was willing to risk it.

I went to church, maybe for the 4th or 5th time in my life. My understanding of spiritual things as a child was that one day I would study world religions and come to a determination of what was true. The idea that God doesn't exist didn't make sense to me because I felt like all of life needed a known human explanation. As a child you don't quite conceptualize that your understanding of the world is severely limited in context with all of the universe and there will always be phenomena we can't account for in the world. The idea that I could even begin to fully understand one religion is ludacris when I look back on it, but you live and you learn. This experience at church was about to introduce me to more unknowns and change the course of my life in a profound way.

Finding God

I went into the small church on a Sunday morning and Karissa's mom was preaching. I had met her mother at the church before, during one of Karissa's classes. She seemed like a nice woman but what I saw that morning elevated her to a different place in my mind. She was charismatic. She weaved together teaching from The Bible and everyday life in a way that was captivating. Pastor Pamela Smith. She was married to the man playing the piano and singing during the service, Pastor William Smith. She preached for about 45 minutes that morning and songs were sung. There was definitely a vibrant energy in that small building that morning.

At the end of her sermon, Pastor Pamela looked at me and she said, "Young man, I don't know you well, but life has been really hard for you. And, it's going to get harder. But God has been with you the whole time. You're going to have a business one day and you are going to minister to lots of people…" There were other things said but this is all I could remember clearly. In particular, the part about life having been hard and it getting harder. First off, this was the first time somebody acknowledged my pain. Even I hadn't verbalized what I had gone through since I was a young boy. Whether it chose me or I chose it, life had been hard for as long as I could remember and up until this point I didn't know that there was something different. However, it tripped me out that things could get harder. In my head I was like, "Harder?! What the Hell?!" Also, I had been thinking more and more about what it might be like to start my own gym. My own business. Somehow, Pastor Pamela was tapping into that thought. She barely knew who I was and I had barely let thoughts of having my own business come out of my mouth to anyone. This was crazy.

I left immediately at the end of the service. On the drive home, I started trying to pick apart what this woman had said to me. There were obvious things that she had touched on that it seemed like no one else could have known. Karissa knew some of my story but not enough to know how difficult it was. I didn't even frame things as having been hard. Life was what it was. I was also numb to it. Hard was normal. Misery was my baseline experience of the world. Being in pain was normal but Pastor Pamela said it out loud and that was not normal. I would never admit such things. I tried to think back on my conversations with Karissa and come up with some sort of way that they were trying to manipulate me but I couldn't find it. It didn't seem logical. If they were running some sort of hustle it couldn't have been bringing in much money because the church was struggling financially. Also, it would have taken a massive amount of energy, effort, and planning to pull off a con, so smoothly. And, even if it was a con, it gave me hope and I desperately needed some hope. I needed someone to see me as I was, not as they wanted me to be.

Hope

Hope is a powerful thing in desperate situations. I started going to church every Sunday. Karissa explained to me that her mom was a prophet, like the ones in the Bible. Whatever energy that was in Pastor Pam that gave her the abilities she had, I was drawn to it. I began reading the Bible everyday and thinking about what I was learning from the stories.

My favorite Biblical Story is the story of Joseph in the Old Testament. The story is told in the Book of Genesis, the first book of The Bible. Joseph was the youngest of 12 brothers who are Sons of Jacob. He has a dream one day that his brothers will bow to him and upon revealing this to his family, his brothers spitefully sold him into slavery. He spends years as a slave to the Egyptians and eventually, due to his diligence in service, he is elevated to a role of Second in Command only to the Pharaoh of Egypt. When famine strikes the land, his brothers must go to the royal courts to get food. They're confronted by an older Joseph who has risen to power but they don't recognize him. Joseph recognizes his brothers and he helps them, though he clearly feels the pain of what they did to him. Eventually, Joseph reveals himself to his brothers and proclaims that God has used his suffering to make him ready to do good for his family and all the people in the land. Joseph's prudence as a slave caused there to be surplus grain during the famine and this helped sustain the kingdom through the drought.

Diligence, suffering, outcast, perseverance, a rise to power, and showing kindness to those who have forsaken you. I felt as though I saw so many parallels to myself in Joseph's story. So many Biblical Movies have been made and I am confused as to how one hasn't been made based on Joseph's story. In the story Joseph says, "What the devil meant for evil, God has turned around and used it for good."

I felt like God was speaking to me through those pages. For a brief time, I began to have greater energy. Karissa and I started dating. My hope was being restored. I felt like the ideas of starting a business that had been in my mind since losing all that weight, were being validated. I would think, "Maybe I can start a business? Maybe I can walk away from Engineering? If I just have faith and trust God, maybe I can do the impossible?"

From late October of 2005 into the New Year of 2006, life was sort of magical. I was dating for the first time ever. I was exploring faith and feeling a sense of hope and joy that could only have been rivaled by how I felt when I was losing weight my senior year in highschool. I was also trying to look at my job differently and be grateful for it. It helped that all new engineers went to Europe for six weeks to participate in a professional development course. I had never been out of the country and I had always wanted to go to Europe. For a moment, things seemed good.

Unraveling

Getting to The Hague in The Netherlands was surreal. The Royal Dutch Shell Company is headquartered there. I arrived along with new engineers to the company from all over the world. That first week, we were given a team building assignment. In groups of about 8 people we were given a small sum of money. We had to get from The Hague to a group of cabins in The Ardennes Mountains in Belgium, south of The Netherlands. Fortunately, there were several people in my group who were native to the area but it was still an adventure. We had to navigate the public transit system and we had missions we had to complete along the way. We had to get random people to let us have a meal in their homes, let us drive their vehicles and even sleep overnight in their homes (that wasn't a part of the assignment but it happened). It was fun!

Once we made it to the cabins we had to do team building exercises. It was cold and snow was everywhere. We had to climb up telephone poles and jump from one to the next, and navigate other physical obstacles. We had to use our brains, our bodies, and we had to work together. It was so much fun. I don't think I had ever had fun like that in my entire life up until that point. It was challenging and frustrating and exhilarating, all at the same time. That first week was amazing. We then returned to the city and this would be the beginning of the end for me.

When we got back to The Hague we began powerpoint classes on the oil and gas industry. It was a basic overview of the entire business. Almost immediately, I was bored out of my mind. From 8am to 5pm we were in class with a 1 hour break for lunch. After about a week of this, I had a nervous breakdown over the phone with my parents. I was screaming at my mother that I wanted to come home. I was hysterical and probably scared the hell out of my family. It was the first time in my life that I was expressing real discontent. More specifically, it was the first time that I was expressing to the world that I was unhappy. It spewed out of me almost uncontrollably.

I managed to calm down after that night but I was definitely losing my grip. During the remainder of the course there were times when other classmates or instructors would ask me how I was enjoying the class. In former years I would have said that everything was fine. However, at this point I would tell the truth. Politely, I would say that I wasn't really enjoying myself. Physiologically, it was as if I couldn't hold it anymore. I got a few light scoldings for my honesty. One instructor said, "You should be grateful! Why are you here if you don't want to be here?!" My parents, Karissa, coworkers, work mentors, everybody was saying this same thing.

As far as my relationship with Karissa, we talked on the phone almost nightly while I was in Europe and we made the decision to commit to one another over the phone. I didn't let her know how miserable I was. I was still reading the Bible regularly and even got into a few religious debates while in Europe. My commitment to Karissa was in many ways also a commitment to faith and sexual abstinence. Pornography was still a large part of my life and something that I used to medicate myself when I was stressed out and, of course, I was stressed out a lot at this point in my life. It was also interesting because Amsterdam was nearby and I visited The Red Light District. It felt like people in Holland were much less restrictive in the way they thought about sexuality. This all juxtaposed to my commitment to faith and abstinence. It was a weird time. Also, there were a couple other female engineers on the trip who were definitely interested in me. One in particular was very aggressive and very attractive. She tried multiple times to get me to come and hang out with her in her hotel room. It was massively tempting. I thought of it as God testing my faith at the time. More than anything, I couldn't live with myself if I lied to Karissa and I valued our relationship too much to give it up for a fling. But I was a virgin and real sex is much more appealing than pornography, at a time where I was finding little enjoyment in anything else. I held on to my faith and didn't go through with anything. Again, it was a weird time.

When I look back, the thing I struggled with most was the feeling like my character was being assaulted by people. By saying that I was being ungrateful for this new job, it felt as though people were calling me lazy and undisciplined. That's how I interpreted it. Here I am saying no to sex with a beautiful woman when I have been craving sex forever. This, after spending my college years with my head buried in a book. And prior to that spending my adolescent years fighting for my health and self-respect. This is all the background stuff that people couldn't see or understand. This was all the hell I had been through and this was what Pastor Pamela acknowledged that day in church when she said, "Life has been hard for you." I made it through the training and I tried to keep my frustrations to myself. However, I knew I was going to have to do something and I was beginning to look at what it would take to pay off my student loans and my car loan. I was planning my escape. But things were going to get harder before they got better…

Breakin' Old Habits

I was happy to return from Europe. The trip as a whole was a good experience. However, 5 weeks of PowerPoint classes on a topic that I cared nothing about was mentally exhausting. I just wasn't interested in oil and gas. When I got back, me and Karissa were doing well, initially. I was going to church and getting to know her family. For a few weeks I was okay but then the same sense of anxiousness and cabin fever began to set in as I went to work every day. The same feeling I had both before and while I was in Europe. I was trying hard to be grateful and in my head I had calculated about two years of working to get all my debts paid off. Again, from all angles I was being told that I should be more grateful: Karissa, my roommate James, my parents, other church members, coworkers etc.

I began traveling to South Texas every other week. Eventually I was being pitched the idea of moving to South Texas in the next year or so. I was not interested at all. The trips to George Bush Intercontinental Airport every other week were some of the gloomiest times during this period. When I got to McAllen, I would stay in a hotel and drive out to the gas fields and try to summon the will to be interested in what I was doing. Similar to what I had been doing for almost 2 decades throughout school. One day I was out in the field with a coworker who was trying to explain something about our processing plants and I drifted off into a daydream. He caught me not paying attention and there came this stern rebuke about me *wanting to be there*. Me *wanting* to do this job. Me needing to let go of my dreams and get realistic. Again, I had a good job and I should be grateful. We went back to the field office and he told me I had some thinking to do.

Back in Houston, things were up and down between myself and Karissa. After about 2 months of being back from Europe, I broke up with her. Whenever we were together, there were times when it felt magical. But then there were other times when the relationship literally made me sick to my stomach. It wasn't her. I had something happening inside of me that I didn't fully understand. I was like Dr. Jekyl and Mr. Hyde. I could be very kind to her in one moment and in the next, not want to see her face. I knew something was off but I didn't know what it was. It would be much later in life when I figured it out. At first I thought I needed to be able to date other women. So I broke it off with her. She was mad but she accepted it. The next time I saw her at church she was polite but barely spoke to me. I was sick to my stomach again and I begged her to take me back. She did but the damage had been done. I had difficulty receiving affection. I could control when and where I gave affection but receiving affection was difficult and it frustrated me when Karissa tried to show affection. Sometimes I could just put a smile on my face but other times I just became angry and lashed out.

Also, I was depressed. Going to work everyday was becoming incredibly difficult and some of the main sources of rebuke were Karissa and other church members. Sunday Night became one of the most difficult times of the week. I had the weekend off and I knew I had to go back to 'jail' on Monday Morning. There were a few Sunday Nights where I had nervous breakdowns in front of her. Work felt much like what being in school felt like. Pure drudgery. Naturally, I would often think, "Is my life always going to be like this?" Even the two years I had planned out for paying off debt seemed like forever. I had spent far too much time being unhappy. People would say, "You're never going to be happy all the time!" But should I be unhappy all the time? Reasonably, Karissa had a habit of asking me about my day at work. I never had anything positive to say. She would try to get me to see the bright side but I couldn't get there. Eventually, I asked her to stop asking about my day because it just frustrated me. I figured it was better to avoid the topic.

One day I remember sitting in my car for lunch and I was playing a CD. It was a song on The Notorious BIG's album that had come out in 2005, The Biggie Duets. The song had a verse from Biggie and featured T.I. and Slim Thug (A local Houston Artist). The name of the song was *Breakin' Old Habits*. One of the lines in the hook went:

You got rich and G-Shit still a part of you,

Why?

'Cause breakin old habits so hard to do.

The song was giving words to something I felt but couldn't articulate in the moment. There was something about romance that I didn't like. It took my edge. It softened me. It made me weak and I hadn't been able to overcome all the challenges I had been through by being soft. It was me against the world. Not, me plus 1 against the world. This was the old habit that was so hard to break. It wasn't Karissa, it was me. I called her that day and I can't remember what I said exactly but it was something to the effect of, *'I'm not the good man you think I am'*. I could feel something was wrong with how I was processing our relationship but I was struggling to reconcile the story I had grown up with, with the reality I was living in. This alongside struggling with the story of success I had grown up with and what I was experiencing at work.

Eventually, graduation season came around again. It was around May of 2006. Karissa had struggled financially to make it through college. It had been a long difficult road for her. She was older than me but it took her 9 years to get her degree and she was going to graduate. My stepsister was also graduating at the time, in Georgia. I was going to drive to see the graduation and see my parents. I figured Karissa should come with me. The day of Karissa's graduation I went to the ceremony and later we went to a party that some of her friends threw for her. It was her day but deep in my gut I was struggling with the relationship. It wasn't other women.

We had planned to get on the road the next day and travel to Birmingham. She was going to meet my parents. The thought of being in the car with her for 10 hours terrified me. All I could imagine was snapping at her the whole time and pushing her away from me when she wanted to be close. After her party, we drove to my house because we were going to leave from there the next morning. I broke it off with her in the car. It broke her heart. Till this day, this is probably the worst thing I have ever done to another human being. Probably the most selfish thing I've ever done to another human being. This was her day and I stole it from her.

The next day while I was driving to Birmingham, I was sick to my stomach. "I love her but I don't love her. I love her but the love is taking something from me that I feel vulnerable without. God, I really did something terrible to her..." I was turning into a nervous wreck all the way around. I wanted her back as soon as I let her go. What was wrong with me and why were my emotions so chaotic?

When I got back to Houston I called her everyday for about 2 weeks and she finally picked up the phone. She let me come over and I begged her to take me back. I cried hard. I didn't want to lose her. I was going to get my act together and I wasn't going to lame out on her again. I was going to figure myself out. She forgave me and she took me back... but the damage had been done.

Falling from Grace

I read the Bible daily. I prayed. I talked to God and I asked him why things were still so hard. I grew closer to my faith but I began to fall deep into depression. Again, Sunday nights were the worst. I began to pray about quitting my job. One of the things that seemed to jump out to me in the biblical stories was the idea of a leap of faith. There are times when people have the faith to endure something (like Joseph in Egypt) and there are times when people have the faith to walk away from something (like Abraham leaving his home). I read the Bible diligently and searched myself constantly.

My relationships were beginning to suffer. James began to withdraw from me when Karissa and I started dating. He had been a devout Christian and seemed generally suspicious about the experience I was having at Karissa's church. In the Western Evangelical Christian World, I've come to learn that people are generally biased towards their form of Christianity and don't do well with varied interpretations. My biggest spiritual practice was reading The Bible and doing my best to understand what was being communicated. That in tandem with daily prayer and working to get various forms of sin out of my life. I didn't want to watch pornography anymore. My language was changing. During college I didn't say anything while I watched James play around with women. He wasn't malicious that I could tell but he did seem to play with female's emotions. It always made me uncomfortable but I didn't feel like I had enough experience to say anything. When I started going to Church I challenged him about it. For so long he seemed to know so much about the Bible and Church and I was a curious novice. But now I was reading the Bible for myself and there seemed to be a huge gap between the virtues espoused and the behavior he was keeping. His response to my challenge was to tell me I wasn't a real Christian and I wasn't going to Heaven. Basically, he told me that my faith was a sham. It broke my heart. This was my closest friend and my first real friend. We were like brothers. We lived in the same apartment but, at that point, we stopped talking to each other. We had a couple more months on our apartment lease. After that time was up, we went our separate ways. We haven't talked to each other since (15-16 years ago).

We were into June 2006 and as I would drive to work everyday I began to become more resentful of the car. It was costing me over $500 a month in a car payment, plus insurance, and all the gas. I was becoming more disconnected and checked out at work. I wasn't getting anything done. It was incredibly difficult for me to concentrate. When I first started working at Shell, I would use a strategy of 50 minutes on and 10 minutes up. Work for 50 minutes and get up and walk around the office for 10 minutes. 9-10 months in, I was working for about 10 minutes and walking for 60-90 minutes. Everyday was becoming painful. Every morning before work I would wake up and feel a tightness in my chest. I didn't know what that feeling was then. It felt like I couldn't take in a full breath. It was scary. Eventually, as I was driving to work, I would start to daydream about slipping my new car under one of the many 18-wheelers that rode along the Interstate 10 corridor. I knew that if my car got totaled, my insurance would pay off the balance of my car loan. I also didn't mind the thought of getting seriously injured and not having to go to work. On the worst days I would imagine taking my own life.

Things were bad. I had stopped exercising and I was eating fast food 3-4 times a day. I was gaining weight rapidly. I had probably put on 30-40 lbs since starting the job. I wasn't functioning. I was having insomnia. I was showing up to work later and later, to start the day, because I was often up all night. There were many days where I didn't shower or change clothes. Just show up to work the next day, disheveled, with the same clothes I had on the day before. I was a wreck but I was trying to hide it from everyone as best I could because nobody wanted to hear it. Not Karissa, not James, my friends, my coworkers, my family, Pastor Pamela, no one wanted to hear it. Remember, I was supposed to be grateful. I had a good job. I felt like I couldn't talk to anyone about it. I was just going to get shut down. To not be able to talk freely about this crushing situation with the people closest to me was incredibly isolating.

I Missed My Flight

I was working with another engineer on my projects at work. His name was Tom. He had lots of experience in the oil and gas industry. At one point we needed to fly to Dallas to visit a vendor who was manufacturing a part for our facilities in South Texas. We scheduled the flight for a Monday Morning, very much the same way I would fly to South Texas every other week. Like many nights at that time, I couldn't sleep. I had to be at George Bush Intercontinental Airport at 10 a.m. I was up by 5a.m. It would have taken me at least an hour to drive to the airport. I was up because I never went to sleep. That morning I sat on the side of the bed from 5 a.m. until I got a call from Tom at about 9:15 a.m. He wanted to know where I was. I told him I wasn't coming. I'd spent 4 hours in the quiet of my room staring at the wall as the sun came up. I was done.

I remember doing something similar in college. When I got tired of studying I would sit in my room with the door closed, lights off, and staring into nothing. It was like my brain needed a reboot so I was trying to shut off all outside stimulus. That morning I felt the same way. I was burned out. Tom told me that we would talk when he got back. Another thing that made this time so hard for me was the fact that for the first time in my life, I was not following through on my responsibilities. I was not performing on my job and it wasn't because I couldn't. I just didn't want to. I wasn't interested in the subject matter. I didn't care about the money or the benefits. I remember walking up and down the halls of the buildings and walking past offices and seeing people staring at their computer screens. I don't know if they were happy or not. I just knew that I didn't want to be them. I was miserable and I didn't see the situation getting any better.

Later that week Tom was back in the office and he sat me down to have a conversation about missing the flight. He asked me, "Travis, what's going on?" In that moment I was going from cognitive disconnect to connection. When I was a young man dealing with abuse, teasing, homelife, school, or whatever, I resolved to never show weakness. Never. I cried myself to sleep many times for many reasons but I would never be broken enough to admit something was wrong. Even though I was having nervous breakdowns and suicidal thoughts I wasn't able to confide in anyone. However, this time, I told Tom the truth. I explained to him how depressed I was and the fact that I wasn't functioning. He looked at me and said that he could tell something was wrong even before the trip. He began to explain that my behavior looked similar to his when he first started as an engineer.

Tom explained that he had a promising athletic career in college but he got his wife pregnant towards the end of school. Instead of continuing to pursue athletics, he felt like he should pursue his professional life as an engineer to give his family a secure living. He said, when he started, he worked with a psychiatrist to get some medications that would stabilize his mood. He earnestly told me that while he was grateful for the standard of living he had, every time he went on vacation he watched the calendar in slight trepidation about going back to work. He also told me that he often checked his retirement balance in anticipation of the day he could walk away. Then he said, "Travis, I had a wife and two children to think about. You are in a very different set of circumstances. I'm not telling you what to do but your situation is different." That conversation has always stuck with me because I feel like Tom was brutally honest in a way that made me feel like I wasn't being ungrateful or foolish. He knew exactly what I was going through.

I thought about it over the weekend. That conversation between Tom and myself was incredibly eye opening because it made me feel like I wasn't crazy. I was leaning towards letting go but I wasn't quite sure yet. What I was sure of was that I needed something to change. My depression was getting worse. My relationships were all suffering as I became more of a recluse. And, I was beginning to gain more and more weight.

One Last Try

I was eating fast food several times a day. I wasn't sleeping. My fantasies of hurting myself in a car accident were getting more elaborate. I wasn't talking to people and when I did talk, I was either complaining or talking about things of little consequence. The more I prayed about it, the more I wanted to let go. Then there came a critical stretch of time, maybe about 2-3 weeks. During that time period, everyday, I woke up, I had tension in my chest. Again, it felt like I couldn't take in a full breath. At the time I thought I was going to have a heart attack. Much later on, I realized I was having mild anxiety attacks every morning. It was scary.

I didn't want to go on medications to live my life. I was scared that I was going to have a heart attack at 24 years old. I had gained so much weight that my back was starting to hurt. I wasn't working out anymore. I needed something to shift. At a minimum, I needed to get back into shape and start eating well again. But I also needed to figure out what I was going to do about work. Engineering wasn't going to workout in the long run but what was I going to do? Maybe I could start personal training? As a matter of fact, I knew that my story of weight loss had some resonance in my work environment.

When I was leaving for Europe to do my initial training for Shell, I decided to run a little experiment. On the outside of my office door I left about 50 flyers. The flyers had pictures of me before and after weight loss. Below the picture I briefly talked about my experience and I gave my top 10 tips for weight loss. I had a deep desire to share what I had learned from my experience. One of the things that helped me get through the trip in Europe was getting a couple of emails from people who had gotten the flyer and were inspired by the story. I knew I had something but I still wasn't confident in my ability to start a business. As I was beginning to experience failings in my own health, I knew that the first step was to be true to myself. In the midst of the fog of depression I began to realize that I was about to forfeit all the work I did to gain my health in the name of keeping this *'good job'* that was killing me.

Then I got a crazy idea... "What about Baseball?" I still loved the game and I still felt like I could play at a decent level if given a chance. I know, crazy. I think I was grasping for anything that seemed healthy and made me feel better. I looked up open tryouts for the Houston Astros online. They had one coming up in about 4 weeks from when I got the idea. I figured, "What's the worst that could happen?"

I had 4 weeks to get myself into shape. The fast food and depression had been wreaking havoc on my body. My back and knees hurt all the time and I had gained about 30-40 lbs. I ended up getting a membership at a gym next to my job. It was too hard to get up early before work to workout because of the commute time and because I was depressed out of my mind. I could start going during lunch time. This would give me something to look forward to everyday and a goal to work towards. That few weeks was the best I had since before starting the job. I felt somewhat normal again. I was hopeful again. People thought I was crazy but I didn't care. The tryout came and went horribly. I didn't have a chance but it was nice to dream again. I had to face reality. Getting my life back was going to be hard and quitting the job was the first step of a long journey.

I was scared. I knew I couldn't keep the job. Work felt like I was going to jail everyday. That brief period of getting back in shape for the baseball tryout confirmed to me that my health was more important than a paycheck. I also knew that my personal story had lots of power to impact people. I had learned that from the experiment with the flyers. I even looked into transferring into the corporate wellness program we had onsite. It was going to take at least 2 years to shift into that role. I didn't have that kind of time. I wanted out immediately. I was scared about what was coming financially. Remember, I had a car loan and student loans to deal with. However, I was more afraid of what would happen to my mental and physical health if I stayed. If I quit, I knew I would get no support from anyone that was close to me. I resigned the week after the baseball tryouts.

The Fallout

Initially, there was a huge feeling of relief. Those first couple weeks felt like I had just been released from prison. Of course, before quitting, many people made sure to let me know how disappointed they were. Karissa communicated an apprehension about the decision in her body language. My mother called and said in a loving tone, "Make sure you tell everybody that me and your stepfather don't agree with what you're doing." While it hurt to have people close to me be unsupportive of the decision, I didn't care. I was free and I believed that if these people loved me, they would eventually see things my way. Call it inexperience, but I would come to learn that just because people love you doesn't mean they have to agree with your decision making. Obvious in hindsight, but difficult to accept when your confidence is low and you are unsure about your future.

Karissa had been pressing me to go to the dentist for a while. At that point I hadn't been to the dentist in years. I didn't think much of it. I went to the appointment thinking I would just get a simple cleaning for $50 for being a first time patient. It wasn't going to be that easy. I still had all four of my wisdom teeth and they were rotting in the back of my mouth. The dentist told me that if I didn't get all four removed soon, they could easily form abscesses and I would have to go to the emergency room. I asked him what the process was to remove them. He told me that I would have to be put under gas anesthesia so he could perform oral surgery to extract the teeth. I wouldn't be able to eat solid food for a few days and it would cost a total of about $6,000. I thought, "I do not have $6,000! Why didn't I go to the dentist before I quit the job?!" I didn't have health insurance anymore. I hadn't been to the dentist in 15 years. I thought, "My damn teeth weren't a priority but that stupid ass car was!" I got the surgery and put it all on a credit card... let the financial troubles begin.

I started hustling to try to make something happen. I had gotten on this kick about faith and God being with me as I worked to help people lose weight. I created my own LLC and started advertising personal training services around town. I got business cards made and went and talked to small privately owned gyms around town. I was networking and I attended a few events on corporate wellness initiatives. I was uniquely interested in corporate health and wellness because of the experience I had just been through. When I left Shell there was almost no one who supported the decision but I could always hear an underlying envy of my choice in people's words. After having that one conversation with Tom on his struggles with mental health when he started, I began to wonder how many more people were struggling with the same issue.

My business wasn't getting any traction. I wasn't making any money and my car payment was falling behind. I was still using whatever room I had on credit cards to buy gas and groceries. I was praying and putting myself out there, but things weren't working. I asked Karissa if I could move in with her. She agreed.

We lived together for about 6 months. I don't think another person's words have cut me so deeply. I was in love with her and after screwing up the way I did before, I was committed to making our relationship work in the long run. I even asked her to marry me. She didn't call me names or cuss me out, but whenever we were talking about future plans, she would make remarks about my choices with a tinge of disgust in her voice. Eventually, I couldn't pay my car payment anymore. I decided to voluntarily surrender my car for repossession. I needed that weight off my back and I needed to figure out what I was doing.

'What do you want me to do? Quit my job?!'

'We all can't just walk away from our jobs, Travis!'

'Well, one of us needs to have a car!'

Statements like these would come in the middle of some argument. I had to get out of her apartment if our relationship was going to make it. She had also been suggesting that I go back into engineering. She wanted me to try to get my job back with Shell. I was foolish enough to try and was vehemently denied. I wanted to prove to her that I loved her and after I moved out of her place I kept looking for another engineering job. Her mother was also in my ear. Comments about being ungrateful, foolish, and not following God's Plan were coming from them and my family. In the midst of all that, I was exercising everyday and feeling better. I was happy to not be going to that office everyday and, even though I didn't have any money, I felt free for the first time in my life. The only time I really struggled is when I was trying to justify my decisions to other people.

When I look back at the struggles that Karissa and I had, I truly believe that much of it originated from my breaking things off, twice. She was trying to let it go but I think the emotional blows were just too much. She was also legitimately concerned by my decision making. I gave up all the effort I had poured into engineering. I allowed my credit to go into the toilet. And, I wanted to get married? Of course she was struggling. I found another apartment and moved out in hopes that it might help our communication. Probably a few days after I moved out, we had an explosive fight over the phone and we broke it off for good. Afterwards, I had a few back and forths with her mother, Pastor Pamela. I presume she was just protecting her daughter but those conversations were contentious.

'You know how many people wish they had a good job like you?!'

'You're not gonna blame my daughter or this church for your foolish decisions!'

I was alone. I was in financial ruin. I was heartbroken. But, I was free. It was crazy feeling all those emotions at the same time. Literally, all my close relationships either fell apart or had become very tense. I hated talking to my family members on the phone because they always had something condescending to say to me... but there were still moments of clarity in all of it.

A Confession

It was a chaotic time but I was holding on to the belief that there was a greater plan for my life than what I had experienced as an engineer. However, I've come to learn that one of the key steps of having an impact on the world around you is the ability to notice yourself. I was learning things about myself. Before we broke up, Karissa and I had been having some discussions around my use of pornography. I loved her and I wanted her to be comfortable with me as a man and that meant being honest about my shortcomings. Whenever we talked about my use of porn I could see the distress on her face. To her credit, she was always gentle with me on this issue. She didn't like it and, of course, in the Christian Worldview it wasn't acceptable. But she didn't judge me and encouraged me in my efforts to stop using pornography. I wanted to stop. I wasn't doing it as often as I had in prior points in my life, but it was still present.

The shame and guilt I felt around porn was something that had always been there since I started looking at it as a little kid. I can still remember seeing that first porn magazine at my sister's boyfriend's apartment. The surge of feelings that ran through my body when I saw a naked woman's body was crazy and I had no framework to process it other than masturbation. It's crazy how our body can instinctively know what to do in response to a stimulus while our mind has no real context for what's happening. What's interesting is that I had been masturbating before I discovered porn. I thought about girls in a sexual way probably as early as the first grade. Once porn came into my awareness, it was something I craved as I got older. I think the good fortune for me is that the internet was nowhere near as well developed and accessible as it is now. This was the late eighties. Pornography was something that you had to buy on video tape, at a store you didn't want anybody seeing you walk into.

The other thing I recognized early on is that masturbation was a stress reliever. As I reached my teenage years and got internet access at home, I began looking up pornography more and more. We also had cable TV at home and the big cable stations would show what was considered soft-core pornography at night, on the weekend. The desire to escape what could be the madness at school and the tension at home, gave me more incentive to dive into this world of digitized sex. I have always contended that pornography is like a drug. By the time I was in a relationship with Karissa, there were moments where my care for her and the guilt I felt from religious beliefs, made me feel as though I could quit cold turkey. However, as soon as I got a little stressed out, I fell right back into it.

Then one day my older sister told me something that changed my understanding of my relationship to porn. At that time, we hadn't been as close as we were when I was a kid but she was curious about church and I was proselytizing a lot. She had been a critic of my choice to leave engineering but I expressed to her that my convictions and my faith in God were leading me. She had been coming to church with me for a few weeks when after one particular service, she felt she needed to tell me something. She confessed that she had physically and sexually abused me when I was little. She was crying and I could see how much it hurt her to admit these things. With as much earnestness and love as I could muster, I tried to express to her that I forgave her and still loved her as much as I always had. It was actually a relief. Earlier in the week I had been watching TV and there was a talk show that referenced studies that showed that people who had experienced sexual abuse as children were more likely to engage in the use of pornography. When my sister confessed, a light bulb turned on for me.

I had these weird memories of sexual acts with my sister, but I always thought they were odd dreams that I was having because of my own sexual diviance. I always thought something was utterly wrong with me and that I was literally broken in some way. I also had memories of the physical abuse and I knew that wasn't a dream. On some level my brain had blocked the sexual abuse out. Like much of the stress I experienced as a kid, I thought it was normal. When you don't have anything to compare it to, your normal environment is your normal environment. As a kid my whole world was chaotic and that's why I never talked about it with anyone. I was intimidated by people because that was the pattern I was taught. My sister could snap on me at any moment and my mother could snap on me at any moment and my response had to be submission. I had no power to speak up or defend myself and as I got bigger and older that mentality stayed the same in many ways. Trauma remembers, so when kids bullied me, I backed down. My internal reaction was to shrink. When my sister confessed, things started to become so much more clear about why I was, the way I was. Granted, I still took personal ownership. I was using porn and I was still easily intimidated by people. I had to figure those things out, but it made a huge difference understanding where those behaviors began.

I didn't fully understand everything that I had been through growing up. It was going to take time to unearth the patterns of thinking that had dominated my life up until that point. But I was seeing things about myself that I had never seen before and it was bringing understanding.

A Long Walk

The reaction I got from sharing that flyer on my office door at Shell that outlined my own weight loss journey, was my first taste of what it might be like to have my own business helping others. Like I said, my own challenges with mental health coupled with hearing Tom's story got me interested in Corporate Health and Wellness. Once I was free from the job and had some time to think, I began working on a presentation that would build off of what I had done on that flyer. Basically, I would go more in depth on the 10 tips to weight loss that I had communicated on the flyer. At this point it was August. I was working to get personal training clients and I had given up my car for repossession. I was trying to avoid conversation with family and friends. I was getting lots of push back on my decisions. One thing you don't need when you're trying to start a business is everyone telling you how much of a mistake you've made.

At my old job, I made an agreement with Shell's Health and Wellness Coordinator that I would give a lunch time presentation to employees. The morning of the presentation, I woke up excited and I had practiced my powerpoint multiple times. I was going to ride the city bus back to my old job to give the presentation. I wanted to get there early so I left the house at around 9 a.m. The talk was scheduled for noon. The bus ride would be about a 2 hour trip. When I got to the bus stop, I was on time, but the bus was late. I started walking in the direction that the bus would travel. I was getting a little nervous and I figured I could at least inch my way closer. I got to the next stop and I didn't see anything. I just kept walking. Eventually I got to the point where I realized that either I missed the bus or it wasn't coming. Time was ticking. In my head, this presentation was an opportunity that I couldn't mess up. So, I kept walking. I thought if I pushed my pace, I could get there on time.

On Google Maps the distance is just over 10 miles and would take around 3 and ½ hours to walk. I had to cut that down by an hour. I got myself focused and started pushing. I got to the building with about 30 minutes to spare. During the walk I had an epiphany. People had always been curious about the big secret to weight loss and I had this nice presentation prepared to give them those secrets. Reduce sugar consumption, drink water, eat less fast food, exercise daily, etc. The hidden secrets to weight loss. As I was walking, I realized I was about to tell people 10 things they already knew. What I hadn't thought to tell them was what I was actually exhibiting by making this 10 mile walk: Perseverance. There's your secret.

It dawned on me that the reason I had been successful in my own journey was the fact that I wouldn't give up, no matter how difficult or improbable. I was resilient, determined, relentless, laser focused, resolute, etc. On the walk I realized that most people would have just called the wellness coordinator and canceled the talk. Not me. Because when things get hard, I tend to dig in and fight harder. This is what helped me see breakthrough as a kid. I would have never gotten to that point at the end of highschool where all the stars aligned, if I had the attitude of most people. If I had let the disappointment of all those repeated failures in losing weight discourage me, I wouldn't have hit that magical window of opportunity. If I had let the harassment from peers and the broken heart I always carried as a child... If I had let those things crush my spirit, I would have never established the habits needed to take advantage of that window of opportunity in my senior year of high school. When I delivered the presentation I scrapped the powerpoint and gave an impassioned, impromptu, and imperfect motivational speech on perseverance. This is what helped me lose weight. This is what helped me make that walk. This is what was helping me believe I could recover from this *'fall from grace'* people felt like I was having. I didn't realize it then, but I was experimenting and I had discovered something: I was a good public speaker and I enjoyed getting the chance to inspire others.

When I got feedback from the wellness coordinator he told me that people loved my passion but they also felt I was a little over the top and *'woe is me'*. I probably said a few things I shouldn't have. But, *'woe is me'*? Never. I was authentic. I admitted all the struggles I was currently facing before a crowd of strangers: Financial Struggles, the Depression, the Debt, all of it. I think this is what threw people off. I had one person come up to me afterwards. She had been an administrative assistant on the same floor I worked on. I never knew it when we worked together, but she had been fighting for her life against cancer. She told me, "Travis, when you're fighting for your life you really begin to get clear on what is important and you need to keep putting your message into the world because this is what people need to hear!"

Corporate America had a tidiness to it that wasn't quite ready for the rawness I brought into the office that day. I had a few conversations with former coworkers afterwards and they were also shocked by the financial struggles I was having. I definitely overshared. I think I was having so many revelations at once that it was simply cathartic to get things off of my chest but people who have it all figured out couldn't see it that way. While the talk went well and I got invited back to do a second one, the conversations with former coworkers knocked me back down to earth. Hard, actually. I was moving forward but I felt like my life was crumbling at the same time and talking with two former coworkers really solidified that feeling. One told me I was crazy. The other scolded me for mentioning his name during my presentation. This guy had told me I was crazy for having a dream and I was angry with him. I didn't come intending to use his name but I let my anger get the best of me in the presentation, along with a ton of other emotions. Like I said, it was raw. I'm still remorseful about mentioning that coworker's name. It was messy and I was erratic emotionally and as much as it frustrated me to be called crazy, I was. I was saying and doing things that were somewhat manic during that time. It was a flood of authenticity and it was beautiful and chaotic, at the same time.

I was heavily leaning on my faith as a reason to justify my actions to those who didn't understand them. At this point, it felt like no one understood me. I had a gift in my story but I needed new conditions and new attitudes to surround me if I was going to cultivate it. One thing that became clear later on was that it's a waste of time trying to convince people of what I see in my own mind. It's my vision and my dream. It's up to me to believe in it. No one else. Ownership.

Isolation

I want to emphasize how paradoxical things were in my life at this time. All my close relationships with people seemed to be falling apart. My mental health seemed to be unstable at times. Financially, I was in ruin. My life felt like a wreck in many ways. However, I was also having moments of clarity and discovering things about myself that would later prove to be very important:

'I am a talented public speaker... I have a powerful personal story... I am not afraid to put my whole story in front of people... When I follow my interests, I'm happy...'

These are the things I would think about and pray about.

Eventually, I found myself alone in an apartment. Me and Karissa had broken up abruptly and my relationship to the Church was over. My old coworkers thought I was a crazy person and my mom made sure that I told people that she and my stepfather disagreed with my career decisions. My stepfather gave me a stern scolding over the phone about how I had fallen from grace and was making bad choices. It was so sobering to have people who had always celebrated me for being so responsible, rip me apart for being flaky and irresponsible. I just didn't want to be miserable anymore and it was as if I were a criminal for wanting such a thing. The final conversation I had with Karissa's mother, Pastor Pamela, was the one that truly broke me. I can still remember her words, "God reigns on the just and the unjust...You're not gonna blame my daughter or this church for your foolish decisions!"

I remember getting off the phone with her and breaking into tears, uncontrollably. I layed on my bathroom floor, curled up in the fetal position for an hour sobbing. It felt as though people had thrown me away like I was a piece of garbage. I was exercising the faith to believe that if I went towards my natural talents and interests, I would be more effective in the world. My faith was very practical. In my mind, how would I be an effective representative for God's Love if I was miserable all the time? Furthermore, how far and how much influence was I likely to gain in a corporate environment where I was just showing up and going through the motions everyday. Church people suggested that I just keep working until I got fired and keep my car until it got forcibly repossessed. What?! I had always thought that part of being a Christian was living with a measure of integrity. I wasn't able to hold up my end of the bargain, so I needed to leave the job. I wasn't able to meet the obligations of my car loan, so I needed to give the car back and deal with the penalties. That's how I saw it, but I was made to feel crazy for thinking that way. No, I let people make me feel crazy.

I gave lots of money to that Church. I did so in earnest belief that the freedom I was discovering through my faith in God, was in large part due to Pastor Pamela's work. It really only seemed fair to me that I should support the church as I could. This was one part of what crushed me that night on the bathroom floor. Other people in my life who had nothing to do with the Church had warned me that the Church might be taking advantage of me financially. To be clear, I don't believe this is true, but in that moment, that night in my bathroom, it felt as though I had been squeezed for what I had and thrown out once I had no more. I had no money and I was having nervous breakdowns. That night on the phone, it felt like everyone had been right about the Church and it crushed me. I was alienated from my family and friends. I was alienated from the Church and the woman I loved. I was flat broke and deep in debt. I was left with all the voices in my head echoing all the criticisms and condemnations.

After I stopped crying that night I thought to myself, "I've been through worse and come out better for it." I was right. In many ways my childhood had been much more difficult. Abuse, constant tension at home, bullying all throughout school, constant disappointment and I still figured out how to do something people spend their whole lives trying to do... I lost 100 pounds. Add to that the relentless work output in my academics. I never liked school but I somehow was able to will myself to good grades as an electrical engineer. To this day, when I tell people I have an electrical engineering degree, people's eyes get a little wide. In that moment I realized that if I could get that far under such stressful conditions, what could I do if I pursued a route that I actually wanted to go down. How much more could I get out of myself by listening to my own instincts and pursuing things that were meaningful to me?

True enough, I was in that apartment alone but it ended up being the best thing that could have happened. I didn't have anyone in my ear telling me their opinions about my life. Anyone can go to school and get an engineering degree. All you have to do is put in the work. Anybody can get into better physical shape. All you have to do is put in the work. However, the work is hard. As they say, *'If it was easy, everybody would do it.'* I knew how to put in the work. I knew how to be consistent over the long haul. I just needed to put that energy in the right direction.

As I was having my revelations and gaining clarity, I began to pick up the pieces, literally. My apartment was a mess. There were papers everywhere, spread on the floor. I was frantically searching for work. One day I came in from job searching all day and I realized, "Dude?! This is not how we live! The first thing you need to do is clean up this damn apartment!" Eventually, the stress of it all caught up to me and I got sick. I layed on the floor of my apartment in the closet for about 3 days, after I had cleaned up the place. I was on the floor because I didn't have a bed to sleep on. Again, I felt like so much garbage that had been tossed out. Whether it was true or not is another thing. I needed a clean apartment and I needed that three days of just sleeping. I had been running around like a mad man trying to find work while also trying to keep myself from crying. I had a couple of nervous breakdowns in public. I was embarrassed, afraid, and I felt like I was a crazy person. Maybe everyone was right? After cleaning my apartment and getting three days of rest, I was able to think more clearly and get back to job hunting. It was a lot for a 24 year old to go through, but I knew how resilient I was. I was wounded but not dead.

***Note - I was a member of 2 more Churches for brief periods during the next ten years after the breakup with Karissa. Today, I would call myself agnostic. I just don't spend any time thinking about the existence or non-existence of God. I don't consider myself a spiritual person in any meaningful way. That journey is a story for another book perhaps.

I'm Not Crazy

Initially, I was still holding on to the possibility of getting back with Karissa. She was my first love so I believed it had to work. In my mind, if I could just get another engineering job, I'd be good again. Even though I was getting some clarity, I was still allowing those critical voices to penetrate my thoughts and influence my actions. I still wanted people to approve of my actions. The bullying at school and at home caused me to seek agreement with people. I wasn't good at advocating for my own thoughts and ideas, even though my actions always suggested that I had exceptional ability to follow through on anything I focused on. I believed I needed people's approval but maybe all I needed to do was decide which direction to focus on?

I needed to pay bills so I scrambled to get a new job. It was another engineering job. The company was a local power company in

Houston, CenterPoint Energy. I was an engineer again and my parents were celebrating me again. On day one, I got the same tension in my chest that I had gotten the last few weeks I was working at Shell. Then something special happened. In the first week of the job I met another engineer who had a real estate business he was building on the side. His name was Victor. He took me out on my first field visit. While we were out on the road I mentioned to him that I had an LLC as a personal trainer. He said, "Man hell yeah! If I was you, I'd be renting my own space for a gym and sleeping in the back!"

"I Lost 100 lbs. Naturally.

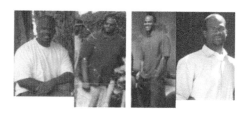

Let Me Train You."

Travis Daigle
Certified Personal Trainer

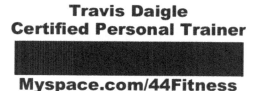

Myspace.com/44Fitness

(Flyer I used for my Personal Training Business. Notice the Myspace. 2007)

HELL! YEAH! This dude got it! He explained to me how he had his own real estate office and had been grinding away at it for several years. He had three kids and a wife and that was primarily why he kept his engineering job. Victor was super encouraging. He even started looking around to try to get me a car. The thing that was so helpful was to know that I wasn't crazy for wanting to do my own thing and walk away from the safe bet. Three weeks into that new job and I was having chest tension everyday. The same tension I had felt just before leaving Shell. I stopped and asked myself a question, "Why am I doing this to myself?" No reason other than pleasing others. I quit.

Engineering was over and I was going to start figuring out how I could make personal training work. I only felt crazy because I kept trying to get validation from other people. I was making the mistake of thinking that I could please myself and everybody else, at the same time. That's not practical. This brief period of time getting to know Victor helped me to realize that. Countless people have left corporate jobs and started businesses. I needed to give being a personal trainer a real shot. Fortunately, there was a major national fitness chain with a location within walking distance from my apartment. I was able to start working there immediately after I left CenterPoint. And, I immediately began to see some faulty assumptions I had made about being a personal trainer.

Fitness Fail

I began shadowing other trainers as they worked with their clients. Salesy, is the word I would use to describe the interactions. Powders, shakes, bars, and wearables were all being upsold to clients. Then there was the entertainment factor. I had one trainer talk to me about keeping things interesting for the client. He talked as he was setting up a mini obstacle course for his next client.

Then there were the clients themselves. The gym was near The Galleria Mall in Houston. It's an area where people have money. High-end housing and sports cars are everywhere. I didn't see determination when these clients walked in the gym. Maybe they needed a friend. Maybe they thought they were ready to do what it takes to lose weight. I was floored by the lackadaisical attitudes. Showing up to sessions late. Making smart-alec remarks in response to corrections on technique. I think what shocked me most about all of this was the fact that I had to learn much of this on my own. These people were paying a hefty dollar just to come into the gym and not take the experts or the process, seriously. It was appalling. I didn't really know what to make of it. The dominant attitudes that people seemed to have towards their own health weren't what I was expecting. This put the trainers in the role of cheerleader rather than fitness expert.

One day I heard a woman say to a trainer, "This is boring! Can't you make it more fun?!" In my head I thought, "What?! You work your ass off now to earn some fun much much later on!!!" I was projecting my experience onto others. I had always assumed that people who hired a personal trainer were doing so because they truly wanted to learn and be pushed to grow. That's not what I was seeing. I wasn't sure what I was witnessing. I would need time to understand what the problem ultimately was.

But I didn't have time. After about 8 weeks of working at the gym, I was running out of money and couldn't pay my rent or my electricity bill. I wasn't picking up any clients. I'm not good at selling things and I'm not a big talker. Especially in new environments. I needed lots of time if I was going to develop those skills. I was short on time. Eventually I got an eviction notice on my front door and that same week the power company turned off my electricity. For two weeks I would come home after work at the gym and sit in a dark empty apartment and contemplate what I was going to do next with my life. It felt like I had truly hit a rock bottom. But I was fine. I didn't have any money but I wasn't miserable anymore. It was weird to be flat broke and totally content with life. I was eating peanut butter and saltine crackers everyday because it was the only thing that I could keep outside of a refrigerator that I could afford. I would charge my cell phone at work each day.

I prayed. I asked God what I should do next. I needed money. I would need much more time to make a liveable wage as a trainer but I didn't have that time. I was getting calls from debt collectors multiple times a day and, of course, I was behind on rent and my electricity bill. It was crazy interacting with the debt collectors. They talked to me as if I was the scum of the earth. It was like I had been going around swiping my credit card on clothes and movies and restaurants. I had to get my rotting wisdom teeth out of my mouth and credit was all I had to do that with.

I meditated and I asked myself very basic, but very important, questions:

1. What do you like doing?
2. What didn't you like about engineering?
3. Where would you like to be 5-7 years from now?
4. What do you need right now?

The answers were simple but powerful:

1. I like being active and using my head.
2. I hated being in an office, behind a computer and I never felt like I had a real purposeful mission as an engineer. It just felt like it was all about making money.
3. I want to be debt free for sure. I'd like to be running my own gym or at least training other people.
4. Right now, I need some money!

At this time I was being extremely logical. I truly believe that my education and experience as an engineer helped me in this moment. I was in what some people might call a mess. I just saw it as a problem that I needed to solve.

One major realization I had during this time in isolation was the fundamental connection between my ability to control my time and my ability to control my spending. Having debt meant that a portion of my future earnings was already spoken for. I had no savings and I was $60,000 in debt. Remember, I needed time at the gym in order to develop the salesmanship skills to build an income. I didn't have that time because I didn't have any savings and I was in debt. I lost the right to experiment with my time because I had been irresponsible with money. Lesson learned. I wasn't going to make that mistake again.

I needed to find a job that gave me an income stream that I could use to begin tackling debt and building some savings. I also needed a job that was more physical and purposeful in nature. I at least had to have a sense that there was real meaning in the job even if other people didn't. Worrying about other people's opinions is what got me into this mess. I wasn't going to make that mistake again.

Again, I was being evicted and the power had been turned off in my apartment. I had done all the crying and being sad that I was going to do. This situation was my doing and I was going to fix it. I was resolute that I would figure things out. I sat calmly at the end of the work day in my dark apartment and I brainstormed. It was cold, rational, logic motivated by a deep determination to do what I wanted to do with my life. No more chasing someone else's vision.

Eventually I thought, "What about the military?"

I Believed a Lie

At the time, the biggest lesson I had learned from losing weight was the value of looking at the truth and taking ownership of that truth. Part of what I realized alone in that apartment was the fact that I had been sold a dream that wasn't reality.

'If you go to college and get a good job you will be successful in life.'

This was the basic narrative that I had been operating under my entire life up until that point. It's a simple statement that makes lots of assumptions. First off, what does the word, *'successful'*, mean? Is it making lots of money? Is it a big house and nice car? Is it being happy? Everyone felt that I was successful because I had gotten an engineering job with a big company. This version of success damn near killed me.

What does it mean to have a good job? Is college the only way to have a good job? These are questions that I never bothered to ask before. I trusted the system I was in. For a brief period of time I was incredibly frustrated. Particularly, as I was getting calls from debt collectors and thinking through how I was going to pay off the $60,000, I kept thinking that someone had done something to me.

I found myself mad at my parents, teachers, friends, family, and the media. "Why did everyone keep telling me to run after this empty promise?!" I may have been in this mindset for about 24 hours and then I said to myself, "Travis, even if everyone conned you and told you something that they knew was a lie, YOU chose to believe it." I looked at the harsh difficult truth and took personal ownership of it. I had gotten myself into a financial mess because I hadn't fully taken responsibility for charting my own course in life. I had spent years killing myself for an engineering degree because I hadn't had the courage to go in the direction that I truly wanted to go in. Those were my choices and my mistakes.

I knew that when I took command I could get a good result. I lost 100 lbs. I also knew that my work ethic was supreme. This wasn't about laziness. I needed to aim my energy in the right direction. But I had to take the time to define the direction I wanted to go in.

For so long, I had been all about the idea of 'never give up'. Now I was beginning to see that there's a time to persevere and there's a time to let go. Basically, I was learning how to quit. When you don't know how to quit, you can end up wasting a lot of time and energy in the wrong direction. Furthermore, I was learning how to envision my future as a whole and work towards that vision. I had done that with weight loss and now I needed to expand that skill to include my whole life.

A Flight Home

I began doing some research online about joining the military. When I was in high school I participated in JROTC. I was encouraged by one of my instructors to consider applying to West Point. He felt I would make a great soldier. I had no interest in joining the military at the time. I didn't like the idea of anyone telling me what to do as I left high school. I was obviously a very self motivated individual. I didn't need anyone looking over my shoulder.

Add to this, September 11, 2001. I had been a Sophomore in my fall semester of college the morning The Twin Towers were attacked in New York City. Being in Houston, I was surrounded by people of all cultures from all around the world. There was immediate violence against people who were from the Middle East. It was disheartening that people's immediate response was bigotry and racism born out of pure fear. The calls for war that came immediately from some of my friends and some voices in the media didn't make sense to me. At that time, as a country, we didn't know what precisely had happened. How were people ready to send military personnel to war within hours of the first plane hitting the World Trade Center? I guess I have always had a tendency to slow down and try to understand what I'm seeing without jumping to conclusions. International issues are obviously complex. I couldn't understand how people were able to justify in their minds violently targeting Middle Eastern or Muslim Students. At the time, I didn't agree with the government's decision to go to war.

Fast forward, as I was contemplating joining the military in 2007, I was thinking about why we had been at war for 6 years at that point. Reports of the deaths of American Service Members in Afghanistan and Iraq were common in the media. Naively, my thought process was that there had to be a just reason as to why we were still engaged in these conflicts. I believed that if I signed up to be a medic, I could focus on saving lives rather than taking them. Again, naive. Also, as a medic I would learn extensively about the human body, knowledge that might come in handy in the future as a gym owner and personal trainer.

In that empty apartment in Houston, I made up my mind that I wanted to join the military. Obviously, being a military medic would be both a physical and mental challenge. It was also a job that had immediate consequences. I could stand in the gap for people who had been injured during combat. I could help save lives. I could have a deep sense of purpose.

My final paycheck from the gym I had been working at was $60. This combined with flight miles that I had collected when I was traveling regularly for Shell, gave me just enough money to buy a one way plane ticket to Birmingham. I got rid of everything I couldn't carry in two bags. One medium sized suitcase and one backpack.

When I got off the plane in Birmingham, my mother met me outside of baggage claim. She told me that I looked like I had just arrived home from a war zone. I hadn't told her about my plans to move forward with the military. I just wanted to get home and go see a recruiter. Visibly, I was pretty beaten down mentally and emotionally. Neither one of us knew how ironic the statement of *'looking like I had been in a war zone'* would become.

PERSONAL OWNERSHIP PRINCIPLE #2:
UNDERSTAND YOUR STORY

Our actions come from our beliefs, even when we don't know what we believe in...

I define the word 'story' as facts weaved together by beliefs/assumptions into a coherent narrative. (I use the words belief and assumption interchangeably) I believe every human being has unconscious beliefs about how life works. The challenge is learning to recognize when our actions are leading us away from our true desires and doing the work to identify the underlying beliefs/assumptions that led us to taking those actions.

If I could've removed the bullying from my K-12 years, obviously it would have been a more pleasant experience. Afterall, my college years were better than my K-12 experience but school was still almost pure drudgery for me. Why? I was never truly interested.

I had a fundamental belief that success looked a specific way. Up until my early 20's, success was master's degree level education or higher. Success involved a relatively high paying job with a well established company. Success involved a certain material standard of living that meant a nice apartment, newer car, and nicer clothes. As a little kid, I can remember seeing the skyscrapers in downtown Houston and dreaming of an office of my own on one of the top floors. Today, the mere thought of working in an office all day is almost painful.

It's not that I have something against education. I actually love learning. It's not that I have something against Corporate America. I benefit on a daily basis from the technology and innovation that comes from large corporations. I'm not against having lots of money or nice things. If these things are deeply meaningful to a person, then they should pursue them. I just realized that they don't mean much to me. My commitment to putting so much effort into this particular version of success came out of a deeply held belief that the college-to-corporate route was the only path to a successful life. Where did this belief come from?

The belief was contained within my overall story about how life works. Life is a broad thing. There's work, personal finances, family, friends, romance, exercising, eating, managing our living space, leisure activity, spiritual activity, and whatever is happening in the rest of the world. Life is really big. I have a theory that we have to make certain assumptions and hold certain beliefs in order to not get overwhelmed by the complexity of it all. How do these stories get formed?

I believe our **Stories originate from Society, Close Relationships, and Self**. When examining your story it helps to focus on a specific area of life. During this time of my life I was wrestling with stories around money, health, family/friends, romance, spirituality, etc. However, the primary source of upheaval in my life centered around my definition of success as it relates to work and career choices.

When I was in that dark apartment facing eviction, the time alone allowed me to reflect on my decisions. I examined my story around a successful career from 3 origins:

- **Society** - A big influence for me was my middle school and high school experiences. These schools were all about getting kids to college. Any prowess in math/science was always held in high regard. There weren't any presentations of alternative routes to meaningful work other than college. I translated that messaging into a very narrow version of success and **I didn't do the work to explore otherwise.**

* **Close Relationships** - If you can remember from the first section, my mother told my sister and I from as early as I can remember that we were poor. She strongly admonished that the way out of poverty was a college degree with academic honors and a high paying job. As far as I could tell, the broader social narrative that I heard in school supported this idea. **Again, I didn't see fit to challenge this idea.**

* **Self** - Ultimately, we're responsible for our interpretation of the world around us. I believe that the experiences of constant ridicule associated with my struggles with obesity caused me to seek the affirmation of others in different ways. As much as I sought isolation when I was young, I wanted to fit in. I didn't enjoy school for a litany of reasons but I cleaved to the approval I got from people when I showed academic prowess. It was the only thing people celebrated me for. This fostered an underlying belief that I needed the approval of other people in order to know I was making the right decisions with my life. That unconscious belief led me to take aggressive action down a path that I didn't really want to go down. **It wasn't until I really scrutinized my story about work and success that I could see the problems in some of my reasoning. I needed to make adjustments.**

There can sometimes be a big difference between what we are confident we can do and what we want to do. The gap between the two offers us the opportunity to engage the process of change. Specifically, changing our beliefs. We act out of our beliefs and our actions have consequences. My actions toward engineering had the consequence of depression, suicidal thoughts, and $60,000 worth of debt. My actions came out of a belief that I needed the approval of romantic partners, family, and friends in terms of life choices. During the time I was working to become an engineer, I shared the same beliefs about success with those individuals close to me but I bore the consequences of those beliefs on my own. Karissa, my parents, Pastor Pam, my friends and former coworkers were not suicidal and deep in debt as a result of my choices. I was. In order to shift my future actions I had to take control of my beliefs and make adjustments based on my own definition of success and my own interests in work. This is really about recognizing when conventional wisdom isn't working for us and being very logical about what we believe will work for us.

We adopt ideas from our surroundings all the time. It's not always a bad thing. I would argue that children need stories because of a lack of experience. I adopted my mother's story on poverty and a successful life. In many ways she was simply communicating the information she believed I needed in order to live a good life. We all have stories and the key is to recognize that life is far too complex for any one person or ideology to accurately tell the story of how the world works. Furthermore, is the recognition that we ourselves as individual human beings are extremely complex and there's a lot we don't know about ourselves. Each one of us has to have the courage and humility to search for the faults in our beliefs and adjust those beliefs when they lead us to actions that take us away from what we truly desire... that's if we are brave enough to acknowledge what we truly desire (this relates to the final principle related to vision).

Once we scrutinize our story and identify problems, we have to begin *asking ourselves what we know to be true* and make reasonable assumptions about the future from there. This is where the connection between the first principle (Action Over Time) connects with this second principle (Understand Your Story). The first personal ownership principle is what allowed me to overcome obesity and earn my engineering degree. What is true about both of these situations? Both situations involved significant goals that took a significant period of time to reach (5+ years each). Both situations involved intensely stressful circumstances. This is true.

With the knowledge that I can overcome difficult circumstances, it now becomes easier to look at the faults in my old beliefs and take ownership of the mess that resulted from those beliefs. In particular, once I'm isolated and not hearing all those negative voices it becomes easier to see the truth. What's happening in my subconscious in this moment of isolation is that my beliefs about myself are shifting because I'm objectively looking at the truth. I had spent so much of my life head down grinding and listening to other people that I never took time to see the relative difficulty of my circumstances and the relative accomplishments. No disrespect intended, but Karissa, my parents, Pastor Pam, my friends and former coworkers had never achieved the things I achieved in the face of the adversity I faced. Furthermore, they're not interested in the things that interest me. Maybe they couldn't overcome being in $60,000 debt but I knew I could. As I wrote earlier:

"I knew that when I took command I could get a good result. I lost 100 lbs. I also knew that my work ethic was supreme. This wasn't about laziness. I needed to aim my energy in the right direction. But I had to take the time to define the direction I wanted to go in."

For so long I didn't have the self-confidence and self-worth to advocate for myself. Ironically, at what most would call my 'lowest point' in life, new self-confidence was beginning to develop. This new confidence was quiet. At the time, I didn't fully have words for the new beliefs I had about myself, I just knew my beliefs were shifting and this is important because *our actions come from our beliefs, even when we don't know what we believe in...*

PART III - VISION

No Rest

The next morning I woke up and I went to my mother and asked for the keys to her car. She wanted to know where I was going. When I told her that I was going to talk to an Army Recruiter, she lost it. Screaming and yelling, she swore that I was going to be forced to sign a contract and sent off to war that day. She cut me down a couple times in that conversation. She insisted that I understand that this wasn't something that I could sign up for and then quit, like I did engineering. Of course, that was still a raw wound for me and she still couldn't understand why I walked away from such a high paying job.

I couldn't understand her either. At the time, it didn't register to me that she might be scared. After all, enlistment at this time was a guarantee that you would go to a combat zone. I hadn't foreseen her fear at all. It wasn't until years later that I could empathize with why my mother was so distraught that day. To an extent, I understood why she was upset but I hadn't really spent any time fully conceptualizing how my decision to join the military felt from her perspective.

"What did she think I was coming home to do? Kick back for a few months and watch TV everyday?" That's what went through my head when we had this moment. I wasn't a *'kick-back and relax'* type of person. I had worked like a mad man losing weight and getting my engineering degree. I was not and I am not, someone who thrives without a challenge in front of me. A big challenge. My parents didn't understand that about me. In no way was it in my mind that it was time to rest. I was in attack mode. I was going to rebuild my life and I was going to be stronger because of everything that had happened. My mind was made.

I got her to calm down and reassured her that I was just going to get information. I went to the recruiter's office.

A Challenge

The Army Recruiter's office was on the Southside of Birmingham not too far from where I went to high school. Initially, I was asked a few questions about my interests. I said I was into fitness and was wondering if I could become an Army Medic. The idea of joining any type of elite unit never crossed my mind. For one, I figured you needed to be in a regular unit for some minimum amount of time before trying out for Special Operations Units. Second, I just didn't see myself as tough enough, smart enough, strong enough, or fast enough to do such a thing. Also, I didn't know how to swim and I was deathly afraid of the water. That's why I didn't consider the Navy or Marines.

Being an Army Medic seemed to be the right fit. Then the recruiter asked if I had a degree. I told him I had a degree in electrical engineering. Then, he asked me something that was going to be life changing, "Have you ever considered trying out for Special Forces?" I said, "I didn't think that was something you could do coming off the street?" He said, "There's a program called The 18 X-Ray Program." It was a bit of a shock to me. I thought, "This guy thinks I should consider trying out for Special Forces?!" I grew up getting picked on for being fat. In my mind, I did not have the skills and toughness needed to do such a thing with any possibility of success. But it did sound intriguing. I told him I needed to do some research and I would be in touch.

Decision Time

I looked into the 18 X-Ray Program. There was a recruiting video online on the Army website. They made it look cool. I read through the training pipeline. A Special Forces Medic takes about 2 years to get through all the training. If I could get through all the phases, I would receive some of the most elite training of any medic throughout all the military services. However, it felt like a long shot and if I failed out I would go to an Infantry Unit. Either way, I was signing up to go to war if I chose this route. I sat and thought about it for about a week. I kept researching. I thought about the consequences. I could die overseas. I could get blown up and disfigured in an IED blast. There were many worst case scenarios. I had to look at the risks with a sober mind because this wasn't a game. Even with the risks and knowing I was unlikely to pass all the training, I decided I wanted to go for it. I figured if I was going to join the Army, why not try to be one of the best soldiers I could possibly be.

When I went back to the recruiters office, he was skeptical. I was concerned. Suddenly he didn't have the same confidence in me that he had before. I think it was because I told him I couldn't swim. He felt as though I should try being a regular soldier first and then try out for Special Forces (SF) later. I agreed. After all, these recruiters were the soldiers. If they felt like I wasn't ready, I assumed there was a good reason they felt that way.

I got everything scheduled to go to the Military Enlistment Processing Station (MEPS) in Montgomery, Alabama. There, I took my physicals and the ASVAB Test. Once I got done with the ASVAB I sat down with a contract specialist to sign my documents and finalize my contract. I was signing up to be what was known as a 68 Whiskey

(68W) or Military Occupational Specialty (MOS), Medic. When I sat down with the contract specialist, he looked at me and told me that he couldn't give me a medic contract. I said, "Why?!" He said, "Your ASVAB score is too high for that son! Do you really want to serve your country?!" I replied, "Of Course I Do!" He said, "Well then you need to sign this Special Forces Contract." I told him I couldn't swim and he responded with reassurance in his voice, "Son, they'll teach you how to swim in basic training." I asked him if I could take some time to think about it. He gave me half a day. I didn't need that long. This was the contract I originally wanted. I took about an hour to think about it and everything in me wanted to go for it.

Upon doing the final contract I was given more news. I knew you could choose to sign up for the US Army GI Bill to go to college but they also had a program that would repay your existing student loans as an alternative to the GI Bill. I chose loan repayment. Being a regular medic came with a $2,000.00 sign on bonus. I thought the SF contract would be the same or nothing at all, since there was no guarantee that I would even pass the selection process to begin the actual training. The contract specialist told me that there was a bonus of $38,000.00 to be distributed in three payments over the first three years of my 5 year contract. I was floored, "WHAT?!" The student loan repayment combined with the bonus was enough money to pay off all my debts. It felt like a miracle.

Basic Training

I was a soldier in Bravo Company 2/54 on Sandhill at Fort Benning, Georgia. I was a member of 3rd Platoon. There were about 40 to 50 of us. On day one, the drill sergeants were in our faces screaming and yelling. I remember having a moment where I thought, "If this is going to be all about getting yelled at and called names, then this is going to be easy! I've been through way worse!" It was my first realization that maybe I had some tools that would come in handy in this environment.

Basic training was all about indoctrination and stress inoculation. The Drill Sergeants wanted us to get used to sleep deprivation and fatigue. They wanted our feet tougher for road marches with heavy equipment. They wanted us in good shape and they wanted us to understand basic combat tactics. It was annoying most of the time but I understood why it needed to be that way. They were getting us ready to go to combat.

I quickly began to realize that this process wasn't what I thought it was about. Before signing up, I feared I would be far behind the curve as far as physical abilities. Of course I had been someone who worked out regularly, but I assumed it wasn't anything like what I was going to experience in the military. However, this wasn't the case. I wasn't the strongest, nor did I possess the most endurance, I wasn't the smartest either... but I showed up. Just like I showed up for workouts on my own as a kid. As with so many other things in life, I just kept showing up and giving it my all. We had 14 weeks to get through and it was a grinder. There were lots of teenagers and, as an older soldier in his mid 20's, the Drill Sergeants gave me a leadership role early in the process. I really didn't know how to handle it. Obviously, I was never a hugely vocal person and some of these young men were utterly confusing to me. I had a deep sense that some of them were not treating the situation with the seriousness it deserved. I think many of them thought this was going to be like a video game. The immaturity was something that grinded away at me because I couldn't understand it. This combined with being told what you are going to do with every waking hour started to take a toll on my mental state at around the 8th week.

The training was also taking its toll physically. In the military there's this thing we like to call, 'The Crud'. Essentially, all those bodies from different parts of the country come together in an open bay to make these super germs that make everybody sick at some point. I had never been one to slow down when I was sick. However, by week 8, I had been sick for 6-7 weeks straight. I woke up one day and felt like crap. We had to go to the field for training. The combination of being sick for so long, dealing with some serious knuckleheads, wanting to fight the Drill Sergeants, and my mind drifting to and from all the chaos that had just happened before I signed up, had worn me down. I was drained physically, mentally, and emotionally.

I requested to sit out training that day. The head drill sergeant knew something was wrong. I was a solid soldier and this was out of character. He came out of drill sergeant mode and talked to me like a normal person. He asked me about life before the Army. I gave him a brief summary of all the crap that had happened beforehand. He told me something that got my head back in the game, "Listen man, you need to focus on you right now. This time is about you rebuilding who you are. You're going back and forth thinking about people who aren't here and don't matter anymore. Focus on Daigle!" He was right. The Army was my opportunity to serve my country and myself. I got back to training determined to not let those ghosts from the past drag me down anymore. I also got some medicine to help me beat The Crud. This was my time to grow and figure some things out about myself. In hindsight, this moment was extremely powerful. I was breaking down and instead of calling me weak, lazy, or ungrateful, this drill sergeant, this battle hardened combat veteran, this white man who grew up dirt poor (as I found out later), got on my level and lifted me up. My whole childhood I had never experienced something like that. This was something like support from a teammate to get through a difficult time. It was so foreign I was almost embarrassed to acknowledge that I needed it. I was so accustomed to picking myself up, alone. It was a huge help. I went out to training with a renewed energy and focus.

The Aggressive Side

Among many firsts, basic training was the first place I got introduced to mixed martial arts (MMA). They called it combatives but it was really Brazilian Jiu Jitsu and Boxing. The first time we were allowed to grapple, I can remember the rush that went through me. I remember being nervous the first time. Would I be scared and back down like I had done so many times in response to physical confrontation as a kid? No. As a matter of fact, I would say I was discovering quite the opposite. I loved the aggressive side of the whole endeavor. I enjoyed the physical confrontation. Shooting big automatic weapons, blowing things up, and hand-to-hand combat. It was the first time somebody gave me permission to be aggressive.

The first time I got on the mat to grapple, me and another soldier from a different platoon wrestled to a stalemate. It was a back and forth struggle without either one of us being able to get the better of the other man. Later on, one of my bunk mates told me that this young man had been a state level competitive wrestler in high school. He was a little heavier than me and much more experienced. This was a huge confidence builder.

As we finished up basic training I was beginning to feel something different inside myself. Confidence that I had never felt before. Obviously, I had been through many hard things in my life at that point, but a new sense of self-respect was coming about through the military. I didn't want to admit it because it seemed so cliche, but the military was making me a better man.

After graduating basic training I headed straight to Airborne School at Fort Benning, GA. The atmosphere was much more relaxed as compared to basic training. We were going to parachute out of airplanes the same way paratroopers did in WWII. On my first jump I had an opening malfunction. My parachute deployed but didn't open fully. I had what's known as a *'cigarette roll'*. My chute was twisted and I was essentially in free fall. What was so cool about this moment was the fact that I stayed calm and simply followed my training. In response to this type of malfunction you are taught to reach overhead and pull your risers apart while making a bicycling motion with your legs. That's precisely what I did. The parachute opened and I landed safely. It was a complete adrenaline rush. As I said, I stayed calm. You'd hate to need a near death experience to develop confidence in yourself but that's what happened. The military was helping me tap into a different part of my personality and it was empowering.

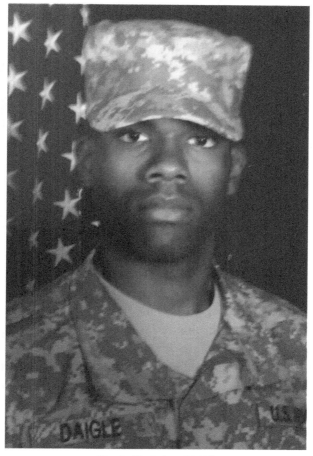

(Basic Training 2007)

Dive In

At the end of Airborne School myself and several other soldiers who had the same contract to try out for Special Forces, were taken aside by the training liaison from Fort Bragg, North Carolina (where the SF Training takes place). SGT Smith had been an Air Force Combat Controller and he had also been to the Army's Combat Diver School in Key West, Florida. It's one of the Army's toughest schools.

Though I was having success in my training up until this point, there was still something that was yet to happen: I still didn't know how to swim and we didn't come close to a pool my entire time in basic training. At one point I asked one of the drill sergeants if we were going to do any water training. He looked at me like I was crazy for asking. There was no water training. During basic training I realized that there were lots of guys who had been given Ranger Contracts and SF Contracts like myself. As I understood it at the time, these were and still are, two of the military's most elite units to be a member of. The best of the best. Many of the recruits who had these contracts were fairly average guys, to include myself. One of my drill sergeants laughed when he found out I had a Special Forces Contract. I guess I didn't fit the part in his mind.

It became clear that some recruiters and contract specialists sold a dream of service to the country in these elite units as a way to get young men to sign up. I want to be clear, it's not all military recruiters. Like any job, there are probably just a handful who don't give a damn. If we failed out of training, it was still a win for them because we would still go on to a regular infantry unit. I don't think any of the recruiters I dealt with saw anything particularly special in me. It was a bit of a let down to realize that my emotions had been manipulated but, nevertheless, I chose to sign the contract. I wasn't going to get help in basic training with swimming, but I could find books on swim technique and I knew all the bases had swimming pools. I could figure it out.

There were five of us whom SGT Smith pulled aside after Airborne School. We were all heading to Fort Bragg, North Carolina. SGT Smith wanted to make sure we had what we needed. He asked, "Is there anyone who has any issues?" I sheepishly raised my hand. He asked me to speak. I replied, "SGT, I don't know how to swim…" He looked at me like I was out of my mind.

He said, "Why did you sign a Special Forces Contract when you don't know how to SWIM?!!"

I replied, "The recruiter told me that I would be taught how to swim in Basic Training…"

His response, "Fuckin' Recruiters!"

He calmed down and looked me in the face and told me to meet him at the pool on Fort Benning, the next day.

The next day came and when it was time to meet SGT Smith I expected that he would show up ready to get in the pool and show me some swim technique. To be clear, the swim test was relatively easy for SF Qualification. You had to swim 50 meters in a uniform and boots with no assistance. You also had to be able to tread water for about 10 seconds. Easy when you're comfortable in the water. Terrifying when you're not. That was me, terrified. But I was determined to make it happen. After all, I was there to become a Special Forces Soldier (AKA - Green Beret).

My fear of the water was multifaceted. By the time I joined the Army, I had never been in water deeper than waist high, other than one incident when I was little. When I was maybe 6-7 years old, I got pushed into a pool by another kid. This was the pool at our apartment complex in Houston. I remember the feeling of gasping for air, sucking in water, flailing in panic, and trying desperately to reach the side of the pool. Fortunately, I got out okay but the incident left an impression in my memory. It was one of the most terrifying things I experienced growing up.

My mother didn't know how to swim and she couldn't afford lessons for me when I was little. By the time we got to Birmingham, my awareness of my body had grown to a point where I tried my best to avoid situations where I had to be shirtless around others. I had bad gynecomastia growing up. For those of you who don't know what that is, it's man boobs. I don't know how else to describe it. Growing up, I got so much grief behind the shape of my chest. It was horrible. I hated it. These two factors meant I avoided the water at all costs.

Now, here I was, a grown man trying out for an elite military unit and I still felt like a scared little kid when I was around swimming pools. A buddy came along with me as moral support the day I met SGT Smith at the pool. He was a stud. He had a Ranger Contract. He had been to a Military Academy for college and I knew that he wasn't one of those accidental recruits like myself. Dude was a savage.

SGT Smith showed up to the pool dressed in his normal uniform and I was a bit confused. He told me to follow him. We walked into the pool area and he walked towards a locker on the side of the pool. He opened it and pulled out a blue brick. He threw the brick into the 15 foot deep end of the pool. My stomach started to turn.

He said to me simply, "Daigle, we don't have time. We don't have time to take you to the kiddie pool and work you up slowly. You've got to go far, fast. Today is all about building confidence. You're scared of the water right now and we need to begin breaking that fear. All you have to do is dive into the pool, hands clasped overhead like a spear. You'll go straight to the bottom. When you get there, grab the brick, squat on the bottom and push off with the brick overhead. You'll float right up."

I was scared as hell and he must have seen it on my face.

He looked at me again, "Daigle, somebody has to go in there and get that brick and it ain't gonna be me. Now, it would be a damn shame if I had to go and ask that young lady over there to come get this brick off the bottom of the pool because your big barrel-chested-freedom-fightin' ass was too scared to do it..." He was referring to the lifeguard on duty. She was probably 20 years old and weighed 110 lbs soaking wet. He was definitely pushing my buttons.

I turned away from the pool and said a little prayer. I also did some risk calculation. If something happened, I had three very water competent people who could dive in the water and come get me before things got bad. I had a lifeguard, a future Army Ranger, and a Combat Diver at the ready if something went wrong. I also thought about how much hell I had gone through before joining the military. At that moment I thought about all the nay-saying people who felt I was so foolish for quitting engineering and every classmate who had treated me like garbage growing up. I needed fuel and I reached into my bag of trauma to find it. Then I thought about what SGT Smith said, "Spear down to the bottom, squat and push off, and you'll float right on up." I thought about that drill sergeant laughing when he found out I had an SF contract and I thought about the contract specialist who lied to me about being taught how to swim. Then I thought, "They don't know who the fuck they're dealing with!" I turned and I dove into the pool head long just like SGT Smith instructed. I got the brick off the bottom of the pool and floated back up and put it at SGT Smith's feet.

As I came out of the water I was flooded with an overwhelming sense of accomplishment. Both my buddy the Ranger and SGT Smith had surprised looks on their faces. My buddy told me, "Travis, they make movies about stuff like this!" We laughed at that one. SGT Smith told me that I had done a good job and that I would be fine in the course. Later on he would tell me that he didn't have a clue how he was going to help me that day and he literally made up that exercise on the spot. He had no idea how I would respond to it. He was surprised that I went after it like that.

That day at the pool proved to be a huge turning point in how I looked at the whole process. I had toughed it out in Basic Training and Airborne School without a problem, but this was different. I had just overcome a massive fear. Mentally, I showed myself to be tougher and stronger than even I thought possible. It seemed like my self-perception was evolving daily. Remember, I thought SF was more well suited to people who had special physical or mental gifts and I saw myself as a long shot to make it. Maybe I wasn't right about that.

Selection

Selection phase is a 2-4 week process that determines which soldiers have what it takes to go on to the Special Forces Qualification Course (SFQC). At that time, all Special Forces (SF) Training was held at Camp McCall near Fort Bragg in North Carolina. The length of the Selection Phase is varied intentionally. The instructors want to keep potential candidates on their toes. Back then, as an 18 X-Ray you were sent to a 4 week prep course after Airborne school. This got you ready to do some of the basic tasks like land navigation and packing your ruck (a large backpack) for long cross country movements. Physically, it was a smoker but it gave guys like me a chance to learn the basic soldiering skills that I didn't have going into selection. Things that I might have learned had I spent time in a regular unit... like climbing a rope.

We had climbed ropes in basic training but I could often get by with using mostly my arms. We weren't climbing super long ropes and the material was something like hemp which meant the grip was good. Not so at SF Selection. During the first event I was faced with a 50 foot rope climb. The rope was nylon which meant it was a bit slippery. Somehow I managed to work my way all the way up to the top using mostly my arms. I wrapped my legs around the rope but I had never learned how to use my feet to clamp down on the rope. At the top there was another rope that we would then shimmy down to get to another obstacle. By the time I got to the top of the 50 foot rope my grip strength was shot. I thought, "Damn! This is just the first obstacle!" My grip was giving out and before I could transition to the next rope, I couldn't hold on any longer.

I didn't let go completely. It was too high. I settled for holding the rope loosely as I sped towards the ground and hit with a fairly loud thud. The cadre (an instructor) asked, "Do you want to carry on candidate?!" I looked at my hands quickly and they were burned raw. All I saw was bright pink patches of raw skin from rope burns. I looked at the instructor and said, "Roger that Sergeant!" I grabbed that rope and made it a third of the way up before my grip gave out again. The instructor allowed me to try once more and then he said, "Get off of my obstacle candidate! Learn how to climb a rope!" I think he wanted me to move on because I started to get blood all over that pretty new white rope.

I finished the rest of the obstacles no problem but I left bloody handprints all over the place. I would do the rest of the 18 days with my hands wrapped up in duct tape and toilet paper from our MRE (packaged meals) rations.

There were other intangible obstacles that went well beyond the course itself. One thing about signing up as an 18 X-ray is the fact that you run into lots of people who have been serving in regular units for multiple years and have multiple combat tours. As an X-ray you're new to the Army and you haven't done anything and there are lots of people who want you to know it. This bothered me. I respect anyone who makes the choice to go and serve their country voluntarily, but not everyone cares to show that same respect in return. Plus there's the whole rank thing. Some people (emphasis on, some) truly felt that because you were of lower rank and hadn't been deployed, you didn't have anything to offer. Then there was the constant alluding that you would crack under the pressure of the training and combat. This frustrated me but it gave me lots of fuel. The more people trash talked, the more I wanted to make them eat their words. If you haven't realized it yet, I'm competitive.

Then there were some black soldiers who swore up and down that white soldiers in the command chain had it out for black guys trying out for SF. Again, emphasis on, some. I ran into three other black soldiers during the selection process. All together, there were a total of 190-200 soldiers trying out, which was a small class. One night during meal time, I ran into two of those other black soldiers and with a small sense of familiarity I asked them if they were ready to attack the next day. Afterall, it was easy to see that there were very few black soldiers in the Special Operations Community. I was looking for that sense of unity and determination in breaking through barriers. The one guy who looked to be the oldest out of the three of us said, "Psshht, we gotta be ready! You know we're the first ones they want to get outta here!" He was smug and very sure of what he was saying. It was as if I had asked a dumb question. I knew what he was actually saying, *'We're black so we are already targeted for elimination because of our skin color.'* Growing up in the South, I knew that tone of voice and look from another black person. It's something that I've never understood.

Are there racists in the military? Hell Yeah! When I graduated from Airborne School, one of the guys I went to basic training with offered to drive me home for Christmas break. A white soldier. He had been in another platoon during basic training. He drove me from North Carolina to Alabama. He came in my house and met my parents. My mother offered to let him and his girlfriend stay at our house and make them breakfast the next morning. When I came back from Christmas leave I found out that he got dropped out of the course because a bunch of Neo-Nazi propaganda was found in his barracks room. Recently, I did a little research and he's been in trouble with the law for hate crimes. As far as I can tell, he's still committed to Neo-Nazi ideology. I don't know what his intention was that night he drove me, but his act was convincing.

Some of my fellow soldiers in basic training had never even seen a black person before. I've always thought of myself as an ambassador for those that look like me. I'll put forth the best effort I can but, racist or not, you will know that you want me at your side when we hit the battlefield. I'm very aware of racism but if my life has shown me anything, it's that people will hate and persecute each other for a litany of reasons. Race is just one of them. I was always aware of the potential of racism but I was careful not to assume anything. I wasn't going to be consumed with fear of something that I couldn't verify was there. Life already had enough real challenges starring me in the face.

Those two black guys ended up quitting. Part of me has always wondered if they were done before they got started. Selection is a game of mental toughness. You don't know how long it will be. You don't know the specific events or their sequence. There are long runs. Hours of physical training meant to take your muscles to failure. There's cross country land navigation. Team events. There are the instructors giving you hell the whole time. In my opinion, there were too many very literal obstacles to deal with, to be worried about whether someone might be racist.

The instructors had the 18 X-Rays help the cadre get equipment issued to the whole class. There were about 15 of us. Alphabetically, my last name was the first among that small group of 15. We also got our roster numbers ahead of the whole class. No one wears rank at SF Selection. Just a roster number. Therefore, of the 190 plus people, I was roster #1, and I heard it every time the instructors saw me. I relished it. Bring it! I've had a target on my back my whole life! There's no way I would have made it if I came predetermined that my being a black man was going to keep me from being successful. I think being black became a barrier for those guys. If anything, I see my skin color as an asset. My ancestors fought for their right to freely and autonomously exist in the world. If they fought, so can I.

Passing this phase of training was another big confidence booster. There were lots of people who ended up quitting or not finishing events. There was one guy in my tent who literally walked the bottoms of his feet off, the same way I had burned my hands raw. The process was going to be tough but I was realizing that I had what it took. It wasn't about athleticism, being the fastest, or being the strongest... It was about mental strength and I seemed to have that in an abundant supply. I was starting to realize that the difficulties I had faced my whole life before the Army had been instrumental in forging the appropriate mindset for the training I was going through.

During Basic Training, Airborne School, Selection, and all of the phases to come, we got pushed to our mental and physical limits. Sleep deprivation, physical exhaustion, lack of mental clarity, hunger, tendonitis, sickness, sprains, strains, and fractures... on top of instructors constantly on your back. It was a grind but it was a grind that I was comfortable with. Dealing with obesity and bullying in school, I understood how to focus on a task in the midst of psychological stress. I understood how to keep getting output from my body even though I was in pain... my knees hurt constantly when I was growing up. Just walking up stairs was challenging to my lungs and my knees. I understood how to focus on complex tasks when tired. My academic work in grade school and especially as an engineering major in college had prepared me for that. I had built all the mental skills needed to thrive in this environment. It's not that things weren't hard for me but I was accustomed to life being hard. Grinding my way through bullies, injuries, disappointment, and tragedy, was familiar.

My Sister

The SFQC (Special Forces Qualification Course) was both challenging and humbling. It took up massive amounts of energy and focus, but the rest of my life didn't stop pushing forward. My sister and I hadn't talked much since I left Houston. She was struggling with bi-polar disorder and she could be incredibly manipulative. It's not that I didn't love her. Quite the contrary. I loved my sister deeply but over the years her behavior had become more erratic and more manipulative. It became difficult to trust her motives for anything. One night I was in my room in the barracks on Ft. Bragg and I woke up in the middle of the night. It was somewhere between 2-3 a.m. I looked at my cell phone. I had a missed call from my stepfather and he had left a voicemail telling me to call home as soon as possible.

I called. My stepfather told me that my sister was dead and had committed suicide. I asked how she did it. He said she put a gun to her head and shot herself. My mother got on the phone. She was crying and her voice was shaky. I forget what we said exactly but I know we said we loved each other and I told her I would be heading that way soon. My initial thoughts were anger. "She quit!!! She Gave up!" Then it was just surreal. I would have these moments where I would say to myself, "My sister isn't here anymore…" It was a crazy feeling but I never could summon the tears to cry. I was grieving but I wasn't devastated. My sister had tried to commit suicide at least one other time to my knowledge and as brilliant as she was, she just wasn't willing to take responsibility for her own choices. Everything that she didn't like about her life was always someone else's fault. This was a big reason we stopped talking. I wouldn't listen to her blame me or our family or her father, anymore. I knew how intelligent she was and she could have done anything she wanted to do. It still makes me sad to think that she couldn't shift into that mindset because she had so much potential. She's still the most intellectually gifted person I've ever known.

After the funeral I came back to Fort Bragg. I had failed the swim test at Selection which was embarrassing but they gave me a second chance before heading out to phase two of training. I had been in the pool on a regular basis getting help from buddies who had been in Navy SEAL training and had been Collegiate swimmers. However, the 10 days away in Houston to attend the funeral had thrown me off and I ended up failing the swim test a second time. After my sister's funeral my mind wasn't focused. Understandably, I suppose. After failing the swim test a second time, I spent some time in my barracks room thinking things over. I remember thinking to myself, "How do I move forward after the loss of my sister?" In some sense, the Army and SF felt a bit insignificant in relation to what had just happened. But like clockwork, another thought entered my head, "You don't honor your sister's life by giving up… You honor her life by getting after it!" I got back in the pool everyday for 6 weeks and I passed the swim test on the third try. I went on to phase two of training with a renewed sense of commitment.

When I failed that second swim test there were a few things happening. Obviously, I had lost my sister. But one of the instructors mentioned something that was becoming more apparent with time. He said, "Daigle, I'm asking you this honestly. We get lots of black guys that come through here and so many of them get bounced by the swim test. Why is that?" I knew he was right but, at the time, I didn't have an answer for him. It wasn't until after I got out of the Army that I met another black, Former Green Beret that I got an idea of what might be happening.

In the mid 20th century blacks were fighting for access. Equal access to education, healthcare, unbiased policing, and... public pools. This other Green Beret told me that he grew up in Colorado in the 70's. His mom took him to the pool once a week at a particular time. He thought that everyone was restricted to that time and day but eventually he came to find out that the time was reserved for black people. After that time passed each week, the city would shut the pool down for cleaning from the *'contamination'*. This was years after the Army that I had this conversation. When my instructor originally asked the question, I told him that my mom didn't know how to swim and pools just weren't easily accessible for me as a kid in Birmingham. But it might be likely that many black men my age have parents who didn't know how to swim. Parents who had grown up in the 50's, 60's, and 70's who may have been restricted from developing the skill and habit of swimming. You can't pass down knowledge that you don't have. This might partially explain why there are so few black men in Military Special Operations. But that's just my own speculation.

Why am I telling you all this? Mental health in the black community is a huge challenge. Mental health problems that we don't talk about. My mom's story of dealing with my sister's drug dealing, physically abusive father and my father, who was mostly absent, is not a unique one. Intense trauma of that sort is common to a lot of black families and other ethnicities as well, including white families. I knew that my becoming a Green Beret was not only a way to build up myself but it was a way to be something representative to other African Americans. Yes we have trauma and lots of adversity in our heritage but it is precisely that adversity that gives us the ability to do really hard things. Moving on with Special Forces Training took on new meaning when my sister passed away. I felt a need to set an example for other black people and really anyone facing any kind of adversity. I felt a need to prove that it was possible to overcome and outlast a difficult past.

Rain

Phase two is the toughest portion of the SFQC. Small Unit Tactics, Land Navigation, and Survival Training are the hallmarks. Navigating the woods with a map was something I experienced for the first time in the military. I was decent but on my first attempt during Selection, I failed due to a stupid mistake. I tried to bust a draw. A draw is a portion of low land that is usually wet and densely vegetated. How dense and how vegetated ranges. We were told never to attempt busting a draw unless we could see through to the other side. On my first point during selection I tried to bust through a thick draw in the middle of the night. Total stupidity. I didn't know what I didn't know. I got stuck in this thing for at least an hour and I got totally turned around once I came out. I had no idea where I was on the map. I walked until daylight came and I hit a major road. Let's just say I was way off course.

My second opportunity to pass land navigation was at the beginning of phase two. I had learned my lesson with the draw but this time I drew a phantom point that several candidates in that class received. Nobody found it. I remember about 5 of us wandering around in the woods in the same area. We looked at each other crazy because we weren't allowed to talk to each other but we all knew we had gotten stumped by the same point. We found out later that the point was difficult to find because it sat in the middle of a draw which made it hard to see once you were within 50 meters. Of course, I wasn't going into any draws because of what happened the first time. However, this time it was daylight and you could see the other side of the draw. I was just gun shy from my previous land navigation experience.

My third and final opportunity came in the middle of phase two between Small Unit Tactics (SUT) and SERE School (SERE - Survival Escape Resistance Evasion). Everyone was going home for a two-day break before SERE School. Those of us who hadn't yet qualified in land navigation would go out with another class beginning their phase two training. This would be our last shot. If I didn't pass, I was out.

They always started us in the middle of the night. Earlier that day one of my instructors for SUT told me that there was a tropical depression moving in off the coast of North Carolina. He said visibility might be tough that night so I needed to make sure I had my head in the game. As we got our point assignments and stepped off, the rain began to drizzle. Moments later it was coming down so hard I could barely see in front of my face. I wore glasses back then and they were totally fogged up. What ensued was some of the heaviest rain I have ever seen in my life. At one point I dropped to a knee because I couldn't see anything. I pulled a poncho over my head to try and get my bearings.

As I kneeled there in the middle of the woods getting what felt like buckets of water dumped on me, I thought to myself, "I guess this is it, I guess I'm out..." My immediate next thought was, "If I'm going out, I'm going out fightin'!" Again, I did what I do. If you hadn't noticed at this point, there is a muscle memory that kicks in for me during these points of intense adversity in life. Unbeknownst to me, it was a mental skill I had developed over the years. Hit a problem, determine my desired outcome, break it down into small steps, and attack. I pulled my map out and under red light checked my route again. I couldn't see, which means I couldn't terrain associate as easily as I normally would. Terrain association is when you translate what you see in land features on the map to what you expect to see on the actual landscape in front of you. I had gotten really good at terrain associating but low visibility meant I couldn't rely heavily on that skill. Just like my instructor warned, visibility was damn near zero. I could take my glasses off, but I was practically blind without them. I would have to rely heavily on the azimuth on my compass for direction and my step count for distance. The absolute basics of land navigation.

For the next few hours I kept my head locked on my compass and diligently kept track of my pace count. I could barely see the end of my outstretched hand. Every time I got to a point where there was a direction change I stopped, got under my poncho, and checked my map again. I was rolling. It was late summer and the rain kept me cool throughout the night to the point that I don't remember stopping to drink water, which is unheard of. I think the rain made me more determined to show what I could do with a compass and a map. I knew I was a good navigator, I had just made a couple of mistakes due to inexperience. Ironically, the first two times I attempted the land navigation courses, the weather was fine. The first time it was a little cold and the second time the weather was perfect. We even had a bright moon in the sky that night on my second attempt.

On this third shot, as I was coming back into the launch area, I was running. I didn't need to. It was just for good measure. I was well ahead of the cut off time and the rain had finally let up. I already knew that there were dudes who just hunkered down all night and didn't try to deal with the rain. As I came in I saw another black guy, Specialist Jason Bates, who I had been in training with. He had gone hard as well. We nodded at each other as if to say, *'Fuck Yeah!'*. We knew what we had done. We both had our best night of land navigation in what were the worst possible conditions. When I turned in my points to the instructor he kind of looked at me the same way the professor in my electromagnetics class did in college when I picked up my final grade. He had that slightly shocked look. He smirked a little and told me, "Good job!" Very few people finished on time that night. Most people didn't finish at all. Understandable... but not me and Jason. Jason went on to become a stud. He went to Ranger School, Combat Diver School, and deployed several times to combat. He had actually overcome drug addiction before joining the Army. Jason was a savage.

Debt Free

The remainder of the course was a series of good moments. After completing phase two, I went on to language school. 6 months of time in the classroom learning Korean. During this time I was allowed to get corrective eye surgery. Up until that point in my life (26 y.o.) I had worn glasses since I was 6 years old for a fairly strong prescription for nearsightedness. I could barely see a foot in front of my face without my glasses. Due to the fact that I had a combat assignment, I had priority to get eye surgery done. It was quick. Two minutes total under the laser and I got out of the chair able to see without my glasses.

During language school I was also able to move into better on-base housing. Up until that point I lived in a barracks building with roommates and a community shower on each floor. I can't tell you how disgusting the bathroom was sometimes. Think about a bunch of early 20 something SF recruits, drinking and partying on the weekends and you can probably imagine. During my training in Korean I was allowed to move into a building that had what were essentially small apartments. I had my own bathroom! Many guys lived off-base but when you are of low rank you don't get a stipend for it. I couldn't afford it because I was kicking out $1200/month paying off debt. I had to live as small as possible.

The last car I had up until this point was the one I gave up for repossession in Houston. I bought a used Nissan from a classmate in my Korean class. It was a 1999 Nissan Altima. It may as well have been a new BMW in my book. It was nice to have more freedom of movement. For that first year or so of being in the Army, I didn't leave the base unless it was with someone else. If you haven't been on a Military base, there isn't much to do or see there. It was a fairly spartan existence compared to most of my fellow soldiers who had houses and nice cars.

When I moved on to the SF Medic Course I was given lots of grief for being one of those people who wore his uniform undershirt out and about in town. I literally had one pair of civilian pants and a couple other civilian shirts. That was it. I didn't really travel anywhere for a long time between having no car and being in and out of the field training. I was laser focused on paying off debt. I barely spent money on anything except the occasional meal at a restaurant or a movie with buddies. I took all my extra money and threw it at my debts. I took my extra time and focused on getting my mind and body ready for training. It was tough, but every month I saw my debt numbers going down and every year we got pay raises in the Army. I began to realize that I could be out of debt two years faster than I originally thought. The more I paid off, the more momentum I got.

Life was good and I was beginning to contemplate what I would do after my first enlistment. During medic training I really got inspired. We were sent on emergency medicine rotations at different hospitals around the country. The medic course was 54 weeks long. During that time you had to complete 2, 1-month rotations at hospitals. 1 in the middle of the course and 1 at the end. I got to do some really cool procedures: I intubated people, helped perform surgery, and I even got to deliver a baby! After my first rotation I thought, "Maybe I should go to medical school?"

However, after my second rotation I began to see a trend that brought me back to the focus I had before joining the military. During both rotations, in two different emergency rooms, it was the same few things that brought people in: chest pain, type 2 diabetes, homelessness, mental health issues, and occasionally, physical trauma. Aside from the trauma and other legitimate chronic challenges, the rest of what I saw probably made up 90% of what came through the ER, both times. Today we call these things lifestyle diseases. I don't remember the doctors using that term but it was clear that most of what we saw originated in people's poor personal habits. I also saw a lot of cynical and burned out medical professionals. I didn't like what I saw overall. I passed on medical school and I'm glad I did. Contrast this with engineering where I had already committed massive amounts of time, energy, and debt into the profession before my first internship. I always tell young people to try to run low cost experiments with career choices. Thankfully, the Army gave me a way to run that experiment with the medical profession while getting paid to do it. I knew I didn't want to do medicine but I still had to figure out if I wanted to stay in the Army or get out and try being a personal trainer, again.

On the whole, life was good. Training was tough but, at this point, I knew I was tough, so it was no big deal. I crushed everything and I took good care of my body as far as I understood how. I was never the most athletic or the smartest, but I was as consistent as it gets.

Once I completed the final phase of training I knew I would be headed to Fort Lewis up in Washington State. It had been a 3 year road by the time I was packing my car to leave North Carolina. I had one final thing I had to do before I cleared Fort Bragg completely. I had to get my security clearance approved. I had only been cleared for an interim security clearance at that point. The debt I was carrying flagged me as a security risk.

Before I went to 1st Special Forces Group at Joint Base Lewis McChord (JBLM), I had to show satisfactory progress in paying off all debts. There was one gentleman I had to check in with who was a civilian and probably retired military. He was my case manager. I still remember that he had a snow-white goatee. I checked in with him three times while I was at Fort Bragg. Once when I first got there, once before heading out to phase two (by this time I had paid maybe $5,000 out of the $60K), and once before leaving. When I showed him that I had a zero balance on all my bills, I got that look again... that same awestruck look I got from my electromagnetics professor, from the instructor at the end of the land navigation course where it rained like hell, and now, this guy.

He was impressed. "You paid off $60K dollars in 3 years?! Good job young man!!" He shook my hand and told me congratulations. He immediately put in the paperwork for my security clearance to be approved. I think he had been accustomed to guys taking forever to pay off small debts. I don't think he had seen someone attack their financial mistakes the way I did, to the level that I did. It was a massively satisfying feeling after everything that had happened before the military.

The breakup, the loss of church community, the claims of being crazy and ungrateful, irresponsible... The calls from the creditors looking to collect debt that I owed... The sitting in that dark apartment where the electricity had been shut off and I was being evicted for failure to pay rent... Here I was three years later completely out of debt, a US Army Green Beret having tackled all the challenges that came with that, I was in great physical shape, and I was confident in myself as a man. If this is what falling from grace meant, then I'll take it... I fell from grace and landed on my feet, stronger than ever. I graduated in the top 20% of my class of Green Beret's and made it to the Commandant's List... I didn't know how to swim when I signed up.

There was a saying that the drill sergeants used often in basic training, *'Improvise, Adapt, and Overcome'*. I had done just that.

Pre Deployment

Once I got to JBLM in Washington State it was like being transported to another world. I had lived in The South my whole life. Now I found myself in what felt like some magical wonderland as I drove into an unfamiliar part of the country, The Pacific Northwest (PNW). It was August. The area was beautiful and the temperature was mild. It was a bit surreal but then I hit the base and very quickly I realized that even in the majestic and beautiful Pacific Northwest, the Army is still the Army and people are still people.

I had gotten done with three years of tough training and making lots of material sacrifices to get out of debt. I was hoping to be able to move off base but I was only an E5 (Sergeant). You had to be one rank higher (E6, Staff Sergeant) to get the housing stipend that would allow me to afford rent in the area. I had spent three years living in barracks rooms and I was over it. One of the big misconceptions people have about the military is the idea that it makes you a disciplined person. In my opinion, it doesn't. What it does is operate on a hierarchical system that punishes those who don't comply. If you already have high levels of discipline and are good at basic things like keeping your living space clean, it's easier to deal with. However, when you're me, you don't like being told what to do or being micromanaged. Constantly being tested and having to prove yourself is another thing that gets old. I thought that this might be a time where I would get a break from the constant assessment but, no such luck.

Right away the other team guys (other Green Berets) are sizing you up and giving you crap because you're an X-Ray and haven't been to combat. Blah Blah Blah... I was happy to be there because I was ready to do the job I had signed up to do. I was ready to do some high quality training with my teammates. I was ready to become proficient with a rifle. I was ready to get into the best shape of my life. I was living in fairy tale land. There was so much paperwork and administrative work that had nothing to do with getting ready to go to combat. Personnel files, making sure people's pay was correct, documentation to account for equipment, powerpoints to explain training plans etc. It was mind numbing. They don't show you any of the constant paperwork in the recruiting videos. To be clear, it's important stuff. I just didn't think paperwork would be a main feature of my job as a medic on a team of Green Berets.

While I hated it, I began to understand the importance of these things as I heard the stories of guys who had gotten injured or killed overseas. There were a few horror stories of spouses that had to struggle to get the support they needed because certain documentation hadn't been done properly before leaving on deployment. The reason this was so specifically impactful on me was the fact that on a Team of Green Beret's the medic is responsible for the basic human resource duties. The junior medic specifically: issues with pay, Wills, Family Medical Leave Act etc. These things fell in my lap without warning. While I understood their importance, I was pissed off. In retrospect I'm glad I didn't know about these things ahead of time because I wouldn't have signed up to try out for SF had I known that administrative duties would be a big part of the job. Every job on the team has its paperwork component. The Engineers who are trained in demolition and construction are also responsible for logging and tracking all of the equipment that a team has. The weapons guys are responsible for keeping track of all weapons systems, ensuring that they get maintenance , and getting range time for the team which is a fairly intense paperwork process. I was not happy with this part of the job but it was critical so I pushed through it.

When I got to my team in October of 2010 we were gearing up to head to Afghanistan. There is a lot to do before heading overseas. Pre-mission Training, gathering intelligence, and understanding the mission objectives. I felt confident in my teammates but my senior medic just happened to be at Combat Dive School when I showed up. Therefore, the responsibility for ensuring that paperwork was done correctly and the responsibility of packing up the needed equipment for Afghanistan was all on the guy who had never been deployed before. I had to figure it out with no experience and little guidance. The rest of my teammates were busy getting their own sections handled and getting affairs with their families squared away. I could have pressed for help but I didn't. However, this was a good learning moment.

What do you do when you are a brand new medic on the team and you have to pack up gear for a year long deployment to a place you've never been to do something you are only familiar with from training? I went to the basics. I packed up things for Emergency Medicine. I packed up things for Clinical Medicine. I packed up things for preventative maintenance. I thought about the basic principles of medicine and combat that I learned from training. I focused on where these areas overlapped. This idea of focusing on basic tasks would come to bear in a very real way in combat.

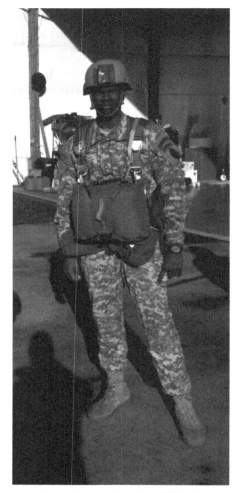

(Jump Day at Fort Lewis 2010)

Afghanistan

Afghanistan was an experience that introduced me to the complexities of war in a way that I couldn't have predicted. By the time I had left training in North Carolina I was fairly certain that the nation's conflicts in Iraq and Afghanistan were much more nuanced and complex than I had seen in the media. There was the collapsing of infrastructure, long standing corruption in government, and the local population trying to live and take care of their families. All this intertwined with terrorists intent to kill Americans. At that point, I'm sure some of those terrorists had adopted their ideology due to actions taken by American Service Members since the wars started. We had been at war for 10 years by the time I stepped foot on Afghan soil. Of course there were Afghans who hated Americans. At the same time, there were locals who loved us because our presence created economic opportunities that they didn't have before. I saw this specifically with the interpreters that my team worked with. Obviously, in some situations interpreters and camp workers proved to be enemies infiltrating American trust. All this to say that my limited experience in Northern Afghanistan makes me fairly certain that I don't understand the full complexity of American involvement in the Middle East. It's complicated. I'm no expert. And, I'm grateful for the experience.

I had been debating whether or not I wanted to stay in the military. The end of the contract I signed was approaching quickly. I was scheduled to either end my service or re-enlist soon after we were scheduled to return from Afghanistan. Deployment would play a huge factor in my decision to leave the military. Yes, the military was full of people who rubbed me the wrong way, but that wasn't the reason I decided to leave.

Once I was on the ground in Afghanistan it became clear to me that understanding the collision of ideologies and cultures that drove the 9/11 attackers wasn't a simple problem. My team was tasked with recruiting and training Afghans to be a police force in their own local villages but there are problems with this that I only see in hindsight:

1. Do we have some common understanding of the rule of law?
2. Do the Afghan People who we encountered in that particular area have the societal will to police themselves into the norms of a social contract that seem stable to us as Americans?
3. Why should Afghans want a social structure that has similarities to that of American Culture?

4. Does our plan truly address meeting basic human needs like food, clean water, safety, and security in a long term sustainable way?

My personal conviction is that stability in Afghanistan has to come from the efforts of those who live there, first and foremost. I believe we got too entrenched in what a vision for a peaceful Afghanistan looks like. Deployment made me realize that I was done. My connection to the mission just wasn't there like I had originally hoped. I thought it better to move on rather than stay and become more cynical than I already was. Midway through my deployment I emailed my chain of command to let them know my intentions were to leave the military.

I was jaded. I just couldn't see the good in what we were doing in Afghanistan or why America had been there for so long at that point. The more I learn about the world, the more I realize how much of a whimsical story I had told myself when signing up for the military. Violent conflict is legitimate at times but it is extraordinarily messy. It brings out the worst and best in humanity. When I signed up to serve, I envisioned chasing the bad guys and going toe-to-toe with evil men. Eventually, a single event summarized the simplicity, complexity, and attractiveness of combat.

Fundamentals Win Fights

One morning we were gearing up for another day of training our local police force whom we had recruited and vetted with local village elders. We had about 200 men from the local area that we trained Monday through Friday in our small camp. I came out towards the group to see one of our interpreters on the phone speaking with a tone of urgency. The sound of gunfire was in the distance... A group of our local trainees were being ambushed. We had to roll out in response.

As we geared up I had one thing on my mind, "I'm knocking some fucking heads off!" I was ready to go to work. This is what I had signed up for. I was ready to prove to myself that I would not be dominated by fear. I was ready to save lives or do my damndest trying. I couldn't think of a better group of guys to go do it with either. We were a rag-tag group of Green Berets and Infantrymen in this remote base in Northern Afghanistan. It was go-time!

Our Fire Base had developed a reputation for being a fairly austere place. We showered out of Camp Showers for quite a while. We ate MRE's. We lived in tents and shipping containers. It was still a lot better than what many service members had experienced in the process of the wars, so I didn't see the big deal. But, it definitely wasn't paradise and I think that created a sense of camaraderie.

As we rolled out of the base in our armored trucks, my mind was thinking through the life threatening injuries I would have to treat as we came on scene. I was trying to get as much information from our interpreter who had been on the phone as I could.

When we arrived on site we linked up with Afghan Police who were already on scene. After my Team Leader got a quick update on the situation, I asked my interpreter to have the police point me towards casualties. He relayed that they had already self-evacuated. In my head I was like, "What?!" There was gunfire, RPG rounds going through the air, mortar rounds etc. And there were no casualties on scene. I thought, "I'm a shooter first! Let's do work!"

Essentially I became another gun in the fight because I wasn't occupied with keeping casualties alive and we didn't have to figure out how to med-evac them off scene. Logistically, it's a lot easier to just focus on wasting your enemy. The beauty of combat in many ways is how singular it is. As the bullets are flying there's only one real response... Fire back.

During the fight we had lots of near misses and bullets whizzing by heads. At one point a mortar round went off right in front of me. It had been placed on a setting where it burrowed into the ground and exploded, rather than exploding in the air. Any shrapnel that could have caused severe damage was suppressed by the Afghan soil.

Initially, our Engineer was in our lead truck trying to operate our 50 Caliber Machine gun. It ran on a remote system where the gunner could be inside the truck operating the weapon, protected from enemy fire. The 50-Caliber Machine Gun is a hallmark of the American Armored Humvee. It's a go-to weapon that we tested everytime we rolled out of the gate. After many successful tests, the first and only time we needed to use the gun in a real situation, it jammed.

I was closest and I was scared because you could hear bullets ricocheting off the truck and going on top of the truck seemed ridiculous at that moment. But, I climbed up there because it was my job. I went through immediate action drills twice with the 50-Cal. The whole time I was praying I wouldn't get shot. Both times the gun didn't respond. I wasn't about to take any more chances so I went into the truck and got our M249 machine gun from behind the front seat. Our Weapons Sergeant had a back up machine gun in each truck.

I went up through the rear hatch on the roof of the truck and started shooting. Long day short, we were on that road all day fighting to include a break mid-day to reload and go right back out. As close as the gunfire and mortar fire was, nobody got hurt. Eventually, we cleared the area and found 15 men dead with their weapons systems that included mortar tubes, Rocket Propelled Grenades (RPG's), AK-47's, and machine guns.

While we were in the fight, we couldn't see where the gun fire was coming from. We only knew that it was one side of the road as opposed to the other and sometimes that didn't even seem right. At one point our Air Force Combat Controller had air assets overhead. An Apache Helicopter made several gun runs on the area in the middle of the fight. The men we found dead in that field didn't stand a chance, but they were close.

In sitting and reviewing what happened during the firefight lots of different things came out. The thing that was most poignant to me was what had happened to our guys who got ambushed and evacuated themselves. We left a medic at our site to take casualties as they came back. He was an Infantry Medic and he did an excellent job receiving casualties.

During the training my teammates and I facilitated, I had been tasked with teaching our trainees basic combat medicine. It was a daunting task considering it was my first time in combat and I didn't have much in the way of guidance at that point. The locals wouldn't have access to any of the equipment or medical supplies that I typically carried with myself on every mission. I had to train them with the tools they already had, with simple strategies they could remember when under fire.

When I was in medic training one of the first things we learned to do came from Vietnam Era Medicine: Stick's and Rags. I was initially intimidated by the task but I quickly realized that all these guys needed to be able to do was keep someone alive long enough to get to the city. We could teach them that without fancy equipment. With the help of the infantry medic and some of the other infantry guys, we taught the locals to make tourniquets and pressure dressings from their head scarves. We showed them how to check and clear an airway and how to check vital signs. Apparently, when those guys self-evacuated back to our site, the infantry medic said they had used some of the methods we taught them.

Basic emergency medicine gave them the ability to take care of themselves. This, of course, was the whole thrust of our mission in Afghanistan. Had they still been there trying to stabilize casualties I would have been occupied with them. Which would have left my teammates with one less gun in the fight. We had two medics die on that deployment from other teams in my company. Oftentimes, medics get shot rendering aid to a wounded soldier. As many close calls as I had that day, I can't imagine how the scenario would have been different if those guys hadn't patched themselves up with what they were taught.

There was nothing sexy or over the top about it. I'm not superman and I'm not a genius. Simple tactics executed well, kept us alive that day.

An International Incident

In the time I've had to reflect on what happened in the gun battle that day I've taken the strategic lessons and tried to put them in practice in all areas of my life. I have also looked back into my life before the military and seen the same lesson playing out in other challenging tasks. Fundamentals win fights. It's the simple things done well that create big changes. This had been a good realization but war also showed me something that is paradoxical about the world.

The day of the gunfight, once the battle was over, we pulled 15 men out of the tall grass along a dirt road in Northern Afghanistan. We were near the city of Kunduz. It's not what we would consider modern by American Standards. By my observation, many people lived a basic life of farming and raising animals for food. No running water available for many people and no electricity. Local strongmen seemed to hold power along with the corrupt government officials they often worked with.

The camp workers who did the jobs available on American bases made themselves a target in many ways. However, the amount of opportunity to create economic mobility for one's self is fairly limited based on what I saw. God forbid you are a woman. The threat of religious fundamentalists who want to keep women from learning or being seen with their faces showing in public is something that I found particularly egregious.

I remember standing on security in one of our guard towers and I would often watch the locals walk by. During the winter, people wore sandals and thinly layered clothing under a winter coat, if people were lucky enough to have one. During one summer day, a man came by riding on a donkey with his son. His wife and daughter walked behind him about ten paces. The wife was dressed head to toe, including a burka which covered her face. This type of thing was appalling for me to see at the time but now I recognize that my understanding of other cultures is filtered through my own culture. Some things aren't particularly fair to judge.

There are components of Afghan Culture to which I had a visceral response. For instance, the power differentials that put everyday people at gross disadvantages. The ALP (Afghan Local Police) that we trained ran a spectrum of what we might call moral standards in common American notions. Some of the men truly wanted to serve their community. Some of the men wanted a chance to do a job they could be proud of. Some of the men wanted to use their new position to assert power over other villagers.

We dealt with regular complaints from local civilians of ALP we trained harassing the local population. It was a dog eat dog environment. There was no way to verify who the men were that day who ambushed our ALP trainees. Were they terrorists? Did they have personal conflict with the men they initially attacked? I don't know. What troubles me till this day is to think that it's highly plausible that some of those men may have been there against their own will. Bullied into attacking Americans because if they didn't, their families would be threatened. Who among these dead men had to make the choice between watching their family be killed or, killing Americans and those that work with Americans?

While I was on mid-tour leave, something happened that I was probably very fortunate to have missed. My team leader and team weapons sergeant got into an altercation that became an international incident.

147

One of the ALP commanders that we trained was accused by a local woman of kidnapping her son. The woman said that the boy had been taken and for two weeks the ALP commander that we had trained had the boy chained to a bed and had been sexually assaulting him. The mother told my teammates through an interpreter that when she tried to plead for the boy's freedom the commander had some of his men beat her up and send her away.

My team leader and weapons sergeant confronted the commander about the charges. He laughed because this sort of thing was normal practice. The sex trade of Afghan boys is an old practice in Afghanistan that even has a name, 'bachi bazi', or 'boy play', as I understand it. Young boys are trained to be dancing boys and are sold into the sex slave trade. My team leader and weapons sergeant probably had a total of 6 years of time in the country at war between the two of them. They had seen this type of thing before. They roughed the guy up a bit. The commander complained to his uncle who was a leader in the local government. His uncle went to the American chain of command and complained.

As I came back into the country off of leave, I found out the news. I was outraged that they had taken my team leader and weapons sergeant off the team. They eventually tried to remove both of them from the military. These are some of the best guys I know and I would still go to war with them until this day. The incident ended up being in the national news. I was glad I wasn't there because I truly believe that I would have advocated that we kill the guy. I think I would have wanted to beat him to death. It was enraging the things we had to just stand by and watch sometimes.

My team leader had filed and reported many other issues of child abuse and pedophilia that existed as a common practice in Afghanistan. He was told to move on because the main objective was to control former Taliban strongholds by placing into power the ALP. The ALP who in some cases made themselves into a new version of the Taliban. War is terribly complicated.

In the middle of the deployment the realities of what I was seeing on the ground in Afghanistan led me to a belief that the best thing for me to do when it came time to re-enlist was to get out of the Army. I was disenchanted. These wars didn't seem to make much sense to me. Why had we been in these countries for so long?

Some of the Afghans didn't even know what 9/11 was. I didn't see the point. The mission I was hoping to connect to, wasn't there. At least, not in my experience. I can't say I felt particularly good or bad about what I did in Afghanistan. I'm grateful my teammates and I came out alive. I'm grateful to have had the experience because it truly gave me perspective on how amazing America is as a country and cultural melting pot. We have the rule of law and we have institutions that uphold the rule of law. Yes, it's flawed but it's still potent in creating an atmosphere where people can flourish. We don't fully recognize how good we have it in America.

About 6 months into my deployment I sent an email to my Battalion Sergeant Major (SGM). I had been pulled to my current team from a different Battalion. My goal in sending the email was to notify my SGM back at home as soon as possible so that he wasn't holding any school slots or team slots for me. I had hoped that deployment might give me a different perspective on the military but not so. I thought that maybe I would go to medical school or physical therapy school in the service. I also thought about trying out for the next level up in Special Operations but once I deployed I realized that I wasn't a career soldier. I thought I was doing the right thing by speaking up and I still believe the stand-up thing to do was to let my SGM know what my plans were. When I sent the email I didn't get any response the entire deployment. I knew this meant some friction was waiting on me when I got back to U.S. soil.

Gratitude

When we got back to base on Fort Lewis (JBLM) I had an interesting moment. I had been living on base housing in a barracks room. When we hit American soil I was looking forward to getting into my room and changing out of my uniform and feeling somewhat normal again. I knew there would be no home coming party for me in Washington. Afterall, I didn't have any family there.

When we entered the First Group Compound and got off the bus, I got my gear and went towards my barracks room. I was happy to be home. When I got to my room, my key code wouldn't open the electronic lock on the door. I tried a few times and realized the battery was dead in the mechanism that controlled the lock. Eventually, I was able to get a hold of someone who controlled access to the rooms and he told me it would be about 30-60 minutes before he would show up. I sat outside on my bags and I watched as one guy after another rode away with his girlfriend or wife and kids.

Ever since the breakup with Karissa I had been alone. Being in Special Operations in the Military, you don't come across a lot of females. Also, I'm not a guy who frequents bars or clubs. I had been leading a fairly minimalist lifestyle. The challenge of this is the fact that a man doesn't meet very many women that way. I longed for romance and I was starting to wonder if I would ever find it again when I got stationed in Washington.

Coming home from Afghanistan that day and watching all my fellow soldiers with their significant others was probably one of the loneliest moments of my life. But, I caught myself. I had just deployed for a year and I was coming home to on-base housing where no one saw fit to make sure that our rooms were operational. I had been through on-base shuffling in and out of rooms since I joined the military and what I felt in this moment of isolation was pure confirmation of my instincts about getting out of the Army. I also still hadn't heard a word from my SGM.

I began to reframe the moment. First off, I was home safely and alive. Once I finally got into my room, I got on the phone and called my mother and told her that I had safely made it back to Washington. I had been so scared for her if something were to happen to me overseas. She had just lost her daughter to suicide a couple years prior to me going off to Afghanistan. I was terrified of what it might do to her if I died overseas. The relief it gave me to call her and tell her I was home safe felt amazing!

The next thing I thought about was money. Yes, I had paid off $60,000 of debt before I went off to Afghanistan but I had no bills when I left the country. That means that I banked $60,000 cash while I was deployed for that year. I entered the Army 5 years prior with $60,000 debt and feeling defeated from all the blows I had been dealt by life. Now I was back on American soil with $60,000 cash in the bank. I didn't have any debt and I could do whatever I wanted because my contract was almost up.

Speaking of my contract, I had accumulated all of this paid vacation time over the years I spent training and deployed. In the 5 year time frame of being in the military, I only took vacation during Christmas time when everyone in the military takes vacation time. Because I was paying off debt as quickly as I could, I learned to appreciate life more, right where I was. Therefore, the need to go on trips or vacations was nullified. I had accumulated 120 days of paid time off.

Sitting on my bags watching the other guys roll out with their families, I also realized that by not having a family, I didn't have to deal with the anxiety of how I was going to maintain my family's current standard of living. In conversations with fellow soldiers, I found out that some guys had multiple home mortgages from time spent at different duty stations. On top of that, people had motorcycles, boats, and big Trucks/SUV's to pay for. Financial discipline wasn't a big thing in military culture. People wanted their toys.

I remember having a couple of poignant discussions with fellow soldiers and teammates before coming home. One guy wanted to buy two motorcycles when he came back home. He didn't have a car, but wanted to buy two brand new motorcycles. I tried desperately to convince him not to, but he wouldn't have it. I told another guy that when I got home I was going to get a car for $5,000-6,000 dollars. To be honest, I considered getting a brand new Subaru Legacy, cash. That would be around $30,000, but then I thought, "Travis, that is a gross misuse of your money! Focus on freedom!"

While I sat on those bags and felt alone because I didn't have romance, I also realized that I didn't have anyone to answer to. My choices were my own. I didn't have a wife telling me we needed a house or new cars or new furniture. I didn't have kids to take care of. I could transition out of the military easily because I had been so financially disciplined.

I realized how blessed I was and how grateful I should be. I was gearing up to move on to the next adventure and it felt good.

Confirming What I Already Knew

I finally sat down with my SGM and he gave me a stern talk about how I was taking advantage of the military and how I was trying to use the SF brand to my advantage. He threatened to try to remove my rank, take my long tab (SF designation), and take my vacation time. Here I was being a stand up guy and telling him early, what my intentions were and this was the treatment that I got. Special Operations brands itself as a brotherhood and just like any family, you have people who view honesty and loyalty in very different ways.

I was upset about the SGM's response to my honesty and deep down I felt a sense of betrayal, but I looked at it as confirmation of what I already knew. Of course, I had people who were asking me what I was going to do when I got out of the military. I told people that my intention was to go into personal training and maybe owning my own gym one day. There was all this concern about money and lifestyle, but I didn't care about any of that. I wanted my freedom back.

In many ways, living in the barracks proved to be a huge asset. Human beings are incredibly adaptive organisms. I might be a highly adaptive human. Barracks life by its nature does not leave one the space to accumulate lots of things. Add to that, the fact that I have never been one to want a lot of things. I had just paid off all that debt and spent lots of time in the military contemplating what debt does to a person's options. It's difficult to make time to consciously experiment with various options in life when you are under the pressure of debt.

I learned how to live lean while I was in the Army. I realized that the quality of my relationships and, more importantly, the quality of effort I put into making myself a better man, is what is most important. Things don't bring me much joy, but the freedom to choose what I do with my time does. Whenever people got out of the military there were always these stories about how they had gotten this fancy job or they were going to this graduate degree program. Again, I didn't care about any of that.

I had begun doing Crossfit about two years before getting out of the service. At the time, I was in love with it. I didn't need, nor did I want a fancy job. I had already started coaching a couple of classes a week at a local Crossfit Gym in Tacoma, WA. Despite what that SGM said, I knew I had served well and I was happy to move on. There was a peace to this time in my life as I was transitioning out of the Army. I had been through hell and back multiple times in my life. I was only 30 years old at the time but I had the life experience of a much older man. Once you go through so many challenges, you realize how much value simple things have, like being able to choose what workout you do in the morning, sleeping in a warm space, having a car that's paid for, being able to get a nice cup of coffee in the morning, or simply not being judged... That few months of transition out of the military was a serene time... My active duty contract with the US Army ended in December of 2012.

PERSONAL OWNERSHIP PRINCIPLE #3: MAINTAIN A VISION

The process is more important than the products...

I define a 'vision' as a set of long term goals an individual has for the future. A vision is characterized by being bold, realistic, and holistic. A bold vision forces one to examine themselves regularly. A realistic vision explores the risks associated with pursuing our goals. A holistic vision tries to account for the totality of life. These 3 characteristics produce a process of personal refinement and self-direction that I believe is more important than achieving the goals themselves.

I can't say it enough, the world is complex. The world is filled with options. Especially if you are American. Social conventions are particularly influential when we don't do the work to choose a direction. If you don't intentionally set your own course it's easy to get swept into the ideas and normal behaviors that permeate your environment. This is how I ended up pouring massive amounts of energy into an engineering degree even when I wanted to major in a different academic field.

However, when you have a clear goal for your future and you are committed to making daily decisions in light of that goal, you can transcend your environment. My weightloss journey is a great example of this. Virtually everyone in my immediate and extended family is overweight or obese. There were no examples of fit adults in my home environment. It was communicated to me by various people that I would never lose weight or be in better shape. Add the broader context of living in the South which is infused with a culture of calorie-rich, decadent food. Obesity and accelerated physical decline is the average in my family. But not for me. Why? Laser focus on a goal of who I wanted to be.

Why Bold?

When I say 'bold vision' I believe the individual should set goals that cause some trepidation. I wasn't consciously aware of this concept when I accepted the opportunity to try out for Special Forces, but I was aware of the fact that challenging processes had the effect of making me a better person regardless of outcome. The lesson that I had learned from my experiences with weight loss, sports, and academics was that failure was okay as long as I gave my best effort to succeed. To be clear, I hate losing and the disappointment of failure can be crushing. However, I've found that disappointment gives way to peace of mind when I give my goals a sincere effort. We can pursue easy targets that require minimal effort and low risk but how does this make you better? We don't know what our limits are until we are pushed to them. Special Forces training allowed me to see things about myself that I wouldn't have, had I chosen an easier route in the military.

It's important to understand that 'bold' is subjective. **This characteristic of a vision requires that the individual be honest with themselves about what they want.** For me I knew I wanted to take on a physically and mentally challenging endeavor and Special Forces training provided that process. The big challenge for me was whether or not I would let the events of the past hold me hostage to a particular story:

'You're weak!'
'You're fat!'

'You're making the worst mistake of your life!'
'You're wasting what God has given you!'

One of the things that became clear to me when I was transitioning away from engineering was the fact that if I chose not to follow my own desire then I would regret it for the rest of my life. I think we all carry regrets of some sort but to consciously suppress our true desires in efforts to please others or to avoid failure is the worst kind of regret in my opinion.

Also, being bold doesn't have to mean big or grandiose goals. Being bold can simply mean being honest. Obviously my career path took a drastic change but my material existence became very simple. Till this day, people ask me about walking away from the money that came with being an engineer and if I regret it. I still say that leaving engineering and joining the military was the best decision I ever made. Learning to be frugal and lead a simple lifestyle were important tools in getting out of debt and they continue to be important tools as I manage building a career as a content creator. Given the fact that common notions of success in our society involve large houses, nice cars, and significant salaries, it took some measure of boldness to walk away from those social conventions. It took courage to say that the corporate career and large salary weren't for me when so many people close to me felt these things were the keys to a successful life.

Bold can mean goals of significant magnitude. Bold also means honesty with self and having the courage to present to the world as we believe ourselves to be, even when that choice brings heavy criticism.

Why Realistic?

A 'realistic vision' is primarily about an acknowledgement of risks. Something that proved hugely beneficial when signing up for the military was the fact that I spent time thinking about the worst case scenarios that could happen before I enlisted.

"What if I'm taken as a prisoner of war? What if I get tortured while in captivity? What if I get maimed by an IED blast? How will these things affect my family and my future?"

This prompted me to think through how I was going to mitigate risks in my daily decisions. Ultimately, mitigation looked like taking the training seriously. This is obvious but it's very different from how I approached college and working as an engineer. No one ever posed the questions, "What if you hate your job as an engineer? What if engineering turns out to be the wrong career field for you?"

It's my opinion that every course of action we take in life has trade-offs and every decision has risks involved. Even the simplest of things. I could go to the gym and risk getting seriously injured trying a new exercise. Also, I could avoid exercise totally and risk losing my physical independence early in life. We shouldn't go on a quest for endeavors with zero risks. We should seek to improve our ability to identify and mitigate risks.

Had I been trained and cultured in an environment of risk mitigation, I may have never ended up in the financial mess that I found myself in after leaving engineering. In taking on student loans, in getting a car loan, and in taking on an expensive apartment, I never thought about what might happen if I suddenly didn't have an income. Therefore, I got blindsided by the fall out. Obviously, I worked my way out of the situation but that transition wouldn't have been as difficult as it was had I done some risk mitigation while still in college.

My mindset shifted as I approached leaving the military. I saved money aggressively because I wanted the option to re-enlist or end my time on active duty when my initial contract ended. Financially, the risk was being lulled into a false sense of security by the consistent paycheck that the military provides. I knew many soldiers who wanted to go back to civilian life at the end of a contract but because they had multiple mortgages, car loans, and credit card debt, they felt like they had no other option besides re-enlistment.

I greatly appreciate my time in the service and I appreciate that I was able to leave on my own terms. Doing so was largely predicated upon being 'eyes-wide-open' about the process. Realism and Optimism are not mutually exclusive. As a matter of fact, by being realistic about the risks associated with my goals I am able to create more strategically effective plans. This makes me more optimistic that I can achieve my goals.

Why Holistic?

When I create a vision I like to think in a 5 year timeline. My military contract just happened to be 5 years. The thing I like about this amount of time is the fact that it's long enough for significant changes to take place but it's short enough to visualize and feel tangible. 5 years might seem a bit too long when you first start doing this so choose a timeline that feels right for you. **I organize my vision into what I call four fundamental areas of life: health, personal finance, relationships, and work.**

These four areas represent the things that we will always have to deal with no matter where we find ourselves in life.

- Health - You only get one body so you better take care of it.
- Personal Finance - The way we manage money is directly connected to the number of options we have in how we live on a daily basis.
- Relationships - Human connection and the quality of our relationships might be the most important factor in our daily lives.
- Work - Having activities that we engage in for their own intrinsic value that give us a sense of meaning is incredibly important. This is our work. This is distinct from work that we do for money to pay bills. There's certainly an overlap sometimes but for many people a job is necessary to pay bills which is more related to personal finance.

A holistic vision takes these four fundamental areas of life into account. When I left college I hadn't intentionally thought about personal finance. I didn't think about how getting a car loan might affect my overall mental health when I accepted the reality that I didn't want to be an engineer any longer. This aspect of vision creation is about learning to set goals in context. Every decision I make in one area of life affects the others.

In my choice to pursue military service I was much more intentional. The decision to be a medic had much to do with learning about the human body which would help later on with being a personal trainer. We've already talked about personal finance habits. Cultivating relationships with other soldiers who lived fiscally disciplined and physically healthy lifestyles was also another conscious decision. The choices I made on a daily basis were made with a greater context in mind. Obviously the unpredictable still happened (learning to swim, my sister's death, etc.). However, by thinking holistically I was able to navigate the unpredictable with relative ease.

The Process

It's an interesting and ironic story to be able to talk to people about how the trials and tribulations of my childhood actually prepared me for my service in the military. However, what if I didn't succeed in passing the Special Forces Qualification Course? I knew many soldiers who got injured in random accidents that meant they got dropped from the course. Soldiers who were smarter and tougher than I am. Fate just happened to be on my side in many situations. The most important part of the military for me was not becoming a Special Forces Soldier. It was the things that I learned about myself in the process of becoming an SF Soldier that were most important. Things that I would have learned whether I passed all the phases of the course or not. Realizing that I was mentally tough, recognizing that I needed to learn self-advocacy, seeing the value of an aggressive outlet, etc. These insights into my own personality have proven to be extremely valuable and would be so whether I became a Green Beret or not.

Long term goals help to specify short term actions. A proper vision helps us wake up everyday and answer the question, "What am I going to do today?" The key is not to become married to specific long term outcomes. We can create a vision and influence the future but we can't predict the future. Facing adversity and the limitations of our stories are always factors in this process. This is where the first two principles connect with this third principle. Part of the reason I am able to set long term goals is because I have the courage to invest long term action into an endeavor where the perceived risk of failure is high (principle #1) and I have the humility to recognize that my beliefs about life will sometimes be proven dead wrong (principle #2).

Over the last 6 years in trying to get people to create visions for their lives, I've typically run into one of two types of people: one type of person who is too afraid of failure to set any meaningful goals and the other type of person sets goals but never acknowledges risks. The former is a persistent pessimist and the later is whimsical to a fault. Both miss the point. Both are so focused on the outcome that they miss out on what is most important: gaining knowledge of self. You have to know yourself in order to take control of your actions, beliefs, and direction in life. Vision is about giving direction to the journey we take in life. It's cliche' but, the journey is more important than the destination because what we learn in *the process is more important than the products.*

CONCLUSION

Personal Trainer to Personal Growth

As I coached classes at the Crossfit Gym and began having conversations with clients about lifestyle change, I began to see some issues fairly quickly. I was a student of fitness and I don't see that as a characteristic only required for fitness professionals. If you want to achieve a goal it seems to me like you should want to learn something about the process related to that goal. If you are trying to get in shape you should be willing to learn about how your body works. To me this seems straight forward. But I came to realize that this attitude is rare in people.

Whether the gym or elsewhere, the biggest challenge I had with getting people to understand how to change their body was taking personal ownership of the process. I think a lack of ownership is the biggest problem people face when trying to get healthy. I fundamentally believe that a person can't say they want to change something they are unwilling to learn about. Naturally, as someone who is in good shape, who lost a bunch of weight, and who had been an Army Green Beret, people were constantly asking me the secret to success. "Travis, what's your secret to being in such good shape? How'd you lose all that weight?!"

That first 3 years after leaving the military I thought I needed to give people some profound insight into cultivating good fitness habits. I would work to simplify things for people. I created videos and encouraged people to focus on simple exercises they could do anywhere. I told people to focus on small dietary changes rather than overhauling everything at once. I tried to make things as simple as possible because I knew how difficult change was. But I quickly began to realize that I had taken something for granted. My belief was always that if a goal is important to you, you should be willing to do everything within your power to achieve that goal and fight through whatever obstacles are presented along the way (principle #1). When I first started coaching people in fitness I assumed that people understood this. Lots of people understand the idea in their mind but I ran into very few clients who embodied the idea.

I've talked with people so many times about some fitness goal they had and so many times I have watched people give up 3-4 weeks into the process, if they start at all. In all of these instances people would agree that hard work is important and fighting through adversity is key. However, so many times I watched people be thwarted by the smallest obstacle: boredom, soreness, not enough time etc. Let alone the big life events like a loss of employment, divorce, or death of a loved one.

Even if the individual was willing to work hard in the gym, if that same person is miserable at work everyday, having trouble in their marriage, and drowning in debt, it gets real hard to say no to that bag of chips at the end of the day when you're exhausted and don't want to cook. You can have the best exercise and diet plan in the world, but if your life is on fire it's going to be incredibly hard to implement and sustain habit changes. I can remember having conversations with clients where I told them that they needed to find a different job or that they needed to leave the gym because membership cost was creating financial stress. These conversations are difficult because they force a person to assess beliefs and that can be a massively disorienting process (principle #2). Also, it requires tons of humility and that's hard in a society where everyone likes to look as if they have it all together.

Finally, with no assessment of personal story people fell into a habit of complacency or, sometimes, firefighting as they bounced from one emergency to the next. This is where clients knew they needed a change in their lives as a whole but were unwilling to try and create a vision for the future (principle #3). Again, for those reasons I listed at the end of part 3:

- A fundamental belief that things won't change and attempting to do so will result in disappointment that's too much to handle.
- Or, a fundamental belief that life is bound to change on its own. Hope and whimsy being the primary strategies here.

I've always been the type of person that wants to get to the source of the problem. You can find massive amounts of free information online that will help you get healthy, help you get out of debt, help you find a new job or start a business, and help you repair broken relationships or move past relationships that can't be repaired. I enjoy examining all of these things but no meaningful change will come about for the individual who doesn't exercise personal ownership. I began to realize that I had much more to offer people than fitness routines. I started speaking and sharing my whole journey in May of 2015.

Since then, I've recognized the common thread in many of the challenges we face in life is the difficulty related to change of any kind. It can be changes we need to make to achieve a goal we have or, more commonly, changes we have to make in response to changes in our environment. In either case my position is that we should be navigators of change, rather than subjects to it. We'd rather take personal ownership of the process as opposed to getting pushed around by it. By taking on this mindset of personal ownership I believe we position ourselves to find peace in life no matter what circumstances present themselves. Also, by taking personal ownership we maximize our potential in the world which I believe very much coincides with having peace of mind. I'm convinced that a large part of the lack of peace, anxiety, fear, frustration and bitterness in our current world is very much related to people who have not explored and expressed their potential in life... and on some level they know it and they avoid the feeling of regret by blaming things outside themselves.

Just in 2020-2021 alone we've seen a global pandemic, massive social unrest, economic recession, uniquely chaotic weather patterns, etc. In the last 20 years we've seen the September 11th Terrorists attacks, the ensuing Wars in Afghanistan and Iraq, Hurricane Katrina, 2008 Financial Collapse, and a host of other things that I've forgotten. This is not to mention the unique challenges that exist in the lives of individuals every single day. Clearly, life is filled with adversity. The question is: Will you own it, or Will it own you?

Presently, the thing that hurts me most in life is to watch people waste their talents and potential as they let life push them around and be bullied, just like kids bullied me when I was growing up. The reason this hurts to see is because I'm a human just like you. I bleed. I feel pain. I need food, water, and oxygen to survive. I'm a collection of atoms just like you. Today as a Former Special Forces Soldier and Combat Vet... Today as someone who attends a Mixed Martial Arts Gym regularly in preparation to get in a cage and fight another trained fighter... I remember being a 10 year old kid and being terrified of the other kids at school... I remember the feeling of anxiety on a daily basis growing up... I remember the heartbreak and disappointment that came with failing to lose weight after so many summers of intense effort... I remember feeling like a scared fool when I was $60,000 in debt and being evicted... I'm human and I found a way to make the adversity of my personal life and the adversity from all the global events I named above, work for me by taking *Personal Ownership*. You can have the same mentality, but it's a choice you have to make.

Yes, life is hard. But, we can *Adapt and Overcome.*

ABOUT THE AUTHOR

Travis Daigle is a Writer, Speaker, Special Forces Veteran, Mixed Martial Artist, and Fitness Enthusiast. For more content visit **TravisDaigle.com**

Made in the USA
Las Vegas, NV
05 October 2023

78625509R00095